AMANDA'S
Gift

AMANDA'S
Gift

One Family's Journey Through the Maze of Serious Childhood Illness

Scott Neil MacLellan

Health Awareness Communications
Roswell, Georgia 30075

Although the author and publisher have made every effort to ensure the accuracy and completeness of information contained in this book, we assume no responsibility for errors, inaccuracies, omissions, or any inconsistency herein. Any slights of people, places, or organizations are unintentional.

First printing 1999

ISBN 0-9665271-6-X

LCCN 98-72996

ATTENTION HEALTH ORGANIZATIONS, HOSPITALS, UNIVERSITIES, COLLEGES, AND PROFESSIONAL GROUPS: Quantity discounts are available on bulk purchases of this book for educational purposes. Special books or book excerpts can also be created to fit specific needs. For information, please contact Health Awareness Communications, 215 Spearfield Trace, Roswell, GA 30075.

DEDICATED TO:

Amanda Leigh, for the struggle she has endured so bravely. Sarah, for the amazing grace she shows in supporting her sister. Deborah, for the courage to be strong when giving up would have been so easy. Our family, friends and neighbors who put up with our repeated late night calls for help. (We never would have made it without you!) Countless "strangers" who pray for her endlessly once they hear her story. And mostly, to the Lord our God, who heals all of us both physically and spiritually.

ACKNOWLEDGMENTS

I would like to thank the many, many people who helped me with this book: my wife and children, who put up with me tapping away at the computer at all hours; my extended family, who provided significant support and encouragement during the early stages of the disease; and some close friends who would not let me give up. I'd like to thank John Cabot, not only for his help as my unofficial editor throughout the initial development of my chapters but for being my cheerleader back when the book was just a few notes scribbled on a piece of paper. And my friend Dianne Jamieson, who helped me get my final manuscript into print.

I'd also like to thank some members of the medical community who went above and beyond in treating Amanda. You cared not only about Amanda but about Deborah and me as well. Dr. Mounif El-Youssef, Dr. Peter F. Whitington, Cassandra Smith and Dr. Charles Rubin—each of you touched our hearts, even if you felt our constant frustration instead of our appreciation. Your dedication helped to inspire hope Amanda could be more than just sick—that she could be a normal, happy little girl.

To the many volunteers at the hospital and the terrific foundations that support programs for seriously ill children, I say thank you. Without your help, we might not have found the few morsels of joy that sustained us during the darkest months.

To the many people who prayed for Amanda for years, even though they may have never met her, I will be forever indebted. Without question your prayers got us to where we are today. You are the reason this book could be written.

"This child, who to all the world looked like a breathing skeleton, had a spirit and soul that were alive with incredible love and warmth. At that moment, I began to understand that we are all so much more than our bodies. The body may be temporary, but Spirit is eternal—grander than the body it goes into. I understood this from the eyes and soul of a child."

—Joan Lauren[1]

1. Joan Lauren, "The Eternal Spirit," *Daily Word*, Vol. 134, No. 2, Feb. 1996 p.4.

PREFACE

This book carries a message of hope not despair. As I write this preface, my daughter Amanda is very much alive, now two months past her most recent "terminal" date. This is her fourth brush with death, and I have every confidence she will make it yet again. She turned six last week and for that we will be forever grateful. Her short life stands as a testament to courage, faith, prayer and modern-day miracles.

Miracles, however, do not always come in neat, tidy packages. Amanda's early years have been fraught with more trials than anyone should have to endure in a lifetime. For all this to have happened to a child seems so grossly unfair. To find any meaning amid all the pain and suffering has been an arduous journey of the soul, a pilgrimage that is not yet complete for me and perhaps never will be. Watching my child go through such trauma has changed me forever.

One thing is certain—dealing with a child who is seriously ill changes every dimension of your life. It becomes all-consuming for every member of your family. To this day, Amanda's illness invades every aspect of my life; it casts a shadow over me. But perhaps how we respond to the sickness that consumes us individually and as a family is what makes the difference between life and death—not physical death, but spiritual. I have died many times in the last six years. Given up. Lost hope. Lost faith. Lived only in anger. And to be honest, I may die a few more times before this is all over. Yet from the depths of this tragedy I have begun to find vibrant life in even the most trivial, everyday events. I have begun to view the shadow cast over me not so much as darkness but more like shelter from a very hot sun.

I now look beyond the physical path that leads me to chaos for a more spiritual path that leads me to peace. And it is on this brighter path I am able to find joy in the moment, not just in the hope of things to come. After all, living in the moment is one of the first lessons you learn in a terminal situation. You have to live one day at a time because to plan anything so often leads to disappointment. At times Amanda's worst bouts with illness seemed to directly relate to major decisions my wife, Deborah, and I were making for our future, all of which were put on hold and most of which we still have not addressed. We used to joke we couldn't plan to walk outside or Amanda might get sick again. Eventually the joking stopped because it became almost eerie how closely our planning of anything (even a simple thing like a date) preceded the quick progression of some new health problem.

So how do we separate the physical from the spiritual? Or better yet, how do we integrate the two? Quite honestly, I'm not sure yet. But one of the things I hope to accomplish in this book is to offer at least a few thoughts on how to live day by day and find joy in the midst of seemingly hopeless circumstances. I cannot guarantee our family experience will help you find hope in your own physical or spiritual struggle, since each person must find his or her own path to peace. But perhaps in reading about our family's journey you will find a light illuminating the starting point of the road you must travel.

My path includes a deep faith in God and Jesus Christ, and I will not hide that in my text nor will I force it upon you. Again, you must choose your own course. Other members of my family have found more bitterness with God than peace. That too is part of the path and probably right for them (and perhaps for you) at this time. Suppressed anger is dangerous. I believe God would rather hear you scream at Him than try to hide bitterness in your heart. The time will come for everyone to find His love.

If you are a parent whose child is in the midst of a lengthy illness, much of our story will be familiar to you. But if you have just started, I encourage you to read this text without fear. You will be tempted to worry and become anxious by some of what I describe. You'll start to think of your own child's future and how it might compare to Amanda's circumstances. DON'T DO IT! Just focus on your child and care for him or her one step at a time. *Love your child! It's all you can do. The rest will just drive you crazy.*

If you are a friend or family member, your role is almost as difficult as that of the parent. Attempting to be supportive and "strong" is very stressful, especially if you don't live nearby. I hope this book provides you with the same principles of peace the parents must learn if they are to survive. Remember, you cannot control events either. You must accept the situation and deal with it as best you can. Otherwise, your frustrations will rub off and eventually cause more stress for the parent.

If you are a doctor, nurse or volunteer, I'm hopeful that in reading these pages you will become even more sensitive to the needs of the entire family. We look to you to help us better understand the complexities of modern-day health care and, more often than not, the intricacies of our wounded spirits. You have an awesome responsibility—one I have come to appreciate more every day. In many ways, you are our guide through the maze leading the way to the best path for our little ones.

And now, as we embark on this journey together, I encourage all of you to find a resting place in your heart—a refuge from the storm that batters you each day. A place where you can go and find the joy in life, even when life seems to offer little to be joyful about.

TABLE OF CONTENTS

INTRODUCTION

Amanda was three days old when she spiked her first fever. After a week in the local children's hospital, she was given a clean bill of health and we were free to go. What a relief! It had been a horrible experience but it was over. We walked out into the Atlanta sunshine feeling lucky we lived in America and had access to the best health care in the world. Our daughter had gotten sick, and the doctors had made her better. Little did we know then we were about to embark on a very painful journey. We would discover it was *not* over; in fact the struggle had hardly begun.

We spent the next twenty-two months trying to figure out what was wrong with our little girl. Her ears constantly dripped puss and were subject to chronic infections. She was tired and often listless, with little or no enthusiasm about anything. She had a rash on her head and groin that would not go away, and she was susceptible to every cold or flu around. The doctors, unable to determine a cause, chalked everything up to an unidentifiable and persistent virus.

After a job change brought us to the Chicago suburbs, we found a doctor who had seen this condition before. As it turned out, Amanda had something called Langerhan's cell histiocytosis (LCH or histio). Histio is an extremely rare, sometimes fatal condition where the histiocytes (a normal type of white blood cell) overreact and attack parts of the body. In Amanda's case, it had attacked her ears, skin and liver. Within days of the diagnosis, she had surgery and began eighteen months of chemotherapy.

1

(Although LCH is not cancer, it is treated as aggressively as cancer.) For so long I had wanted to know the nature of my daughter's illness. I thought if we could identify it, we could fight it, fix it, beat it and bring an end to the sickness. But instead, all we had done was to name an elusive demon. The nightmare was not ending, it had only just begun.

In only two years the histio completely destroyed her liver. Facing ultimate organ failure, she received a liver transplant in November 1993. After a couple of bouts of rejection, Amanda seemed to be on her way to recovery. But the same drugs she took to keep her body from rejecting the liver also made her susceptible to cancer. In May 1994 she was diagnosed with lymphoma. A tumor the size of a grapefruit had grown in her chest and was pressing against her heart. Several surgeries and another six months of chemotherapy seemed to get the cancer under control. Once again we thought the most difficult part of the journey was behind us.

In May 1995, however, we discovered although she had been on the chemo for almost a year (as a prevention tool), the cancer had returned, this time much more aggressively. The one tumor in her chest had grown back and extended throughout her body. It had grown down into her belly and created two large masses in her abdomen. It had also grown completely around her heart and through the heart wall to the inside chambers, where it branched off into three more tumors.

Without treatment, doctors said, she would live thirty days; with treatment, they weren't sure. Post-transplant lymphomas are very rare, and little is known about how they react. And if they treated her with ultra-aggressive chemotherapy, it might cause one of the tumors inside her heart to break off and kill her instantly. What to do? For the first time, we seriously considered not treating the disease and letting her die. We had thought about "letting her go" a few times over the years but never for very long. This time, though, she was probably going to die anyway. Why spend the last few weeks of her life in a hospital in pain from the cancer while also dealing with the horrible side effects of chemotherapy? Why not take her home to be in a safe, loving environment when she died?

After three of the most difficult days of our lives, we made a choice. Knowing that with no treatment she would surely die, our choice was to treat it aggressively. The chemotherapy began late on a Friday night. As I watched it go from the IV bag into her tiny body, I was numb. I had no feeling. I just couldn't believe we had come to this point one more time. Yet another fight for life. I sat there wondering if I had any fight left in me. More important, did Amanda? I wondered why our lives couldn't be like other people's. I wondered why it couldn't be me lying in that bed instead of my child. I wondered why God had abandoned our family.

The first few weeks were as bad as expected. After the first five days of treatment, we ended up back in the hospital twice more dealing with the complications of both the chemo and the cancer. Amanda sunk into a state I had never seen before, even during the most challenging times. She was in extreme pain and completely unresponsive. At least twice as I held her in my arms with my wife, Deborah, and my oldest daughter, Sarah, only inches away, I was absolutely certain I was watching Amanda take her last breaths. I was watching my daughter die! I don't think I will ever be able to describe the feeling of watching my daughter die. To put it into words would somehow diminish its significance.

But Amanda found the strength from somewhere to come back from the depths of her illness. Around the third week of treatment she was noticeably different—somehow slightly more energetic, a little more interested in what was happening around her. By week six, the tumors were much smaller and Amanda was playing with friends. It was like watching her be reborn. In many ways, she began to look better than she ever had. Our daughter was back!

Today she is continuing her chemotherapy and is still heading in the right direction. We still don't know what will happen to her six months or a year from now. In order to treat the current cancer, we have had to take her off her antirejection drugs again. We're in a catch-22 situation. When we treat her cancer, her body rejects her liver. When we treat her body's rejection, the cancer takes over. Neither option seems to offer a permanent recovery. For now, all we can do is treat the cancer and hope that somewhere the cycle will break. Somehow this child deserves a chance at life.

In the long run, however, how we define life may end up being the secret to finding joy in seemingly desperate situations. We all have expectations of what our lives should be like; how we should live, how long we should live and under what circumstances. Such expectations play an important part in shaping our everyday hopes and dreams. But if we continually measure our lives against some specific benchmark we have set for ourselves, we will be forever disappointed. The details of our lives will never match exactly to what we have imagined. But the details are not what we're really after. Most of us are after loving relationships, joy, prosperity, abundance, creativity, growth and perhaps faith. And it may just be that somewhere in the details of our tragedy, all of these things exist in perfect harmony. Finding that harmony can be at the heart of our journey.

In the pages that follow, we'll search together for the balance between the joy and the pain, the spirit and the body, our dreams and our realities of everyday life in a hospital. I'll describe our experience with issues that face any family going through the health-care system. Most of these issues will be fact-based, day-to-day details on how to manage through serious illness. Others will be more passionate subjects that get to the emotions behind the experience.

At the beginning of each chapter, I'll share with you a few of my journal entries over the years, which may add more of an emotional perspective on Amanda's story. The chapters will focus more on the issues and objective detail. I hope this information will help each of you as you find your way in caring for your child.

Thank you for choosing this book. I wish you every blessing as your child recovers. Remember to keep the faith. All is not lost.

CHAPTER 1

Entering the Maze of Childhood Illness

"Blessed is a man who perseveres under trial; for once he has been approved, he will receive the crown of life, which the Lord has promised to those who love Him."

—James 1:12

Journal Entry: May 1991

I actually couldn't speak. It was all I could do to breathe. I was the one who had made the phone call, but still I couldn't speak. I was afraid that if I actually said the words, it might be true. The doctor had told me just minutes before. Why had I rushed to tell my parents? I wasn't ready yet. Deborah and I had suspected this news during the two-week wait for the test results, but never really believed it could happen to us. I had accepted the doctor's news with relative grace; almost stone faced. Now in the role of serving as communicator, I was completely unprepared. All at once, I was three years old—wanting to run to my parents and tell them to hold me. I never did that then; why did I want to do it now?

Still unable to speak the words, I couldn't even cry out loud. I can only imagine what they must have been thinking with all the silence on the other end of the phone. And then the tears came. I hadn't cried in front of my parents for years.

7

Even now, on the phone, it felt strange. Finally, I was able to tell them that Amanda had been diagnosed with a rare form of cancer. The conversation was brief and to the point. "I'll call back later. I can't talk about it now. I can't even breathe."

Journal Entry: June 1991

Today we learned that Amanda's illness is not cancer, but a rare disease that is treated like cancer. That was supposed to make me feel better, but I'm not sure if it did. My daughter will never be the same again. How can that make me feel any better?

The "routine" tests felt less than routine. Repeated sticks for blood work, X-rays, ultrasounds and the fourth biopsy of her head rash took six hours. Amanda did not do well. She was hysterical and we had to hold her down through most of the procedures. Her screams were painful for Deborah and me, but even worse were the few times she was silent. She stared at us with curiosity as to why we were participating in all this cruelty. Her trust in us diminished by the hour.

For some reason, they kept taking photographs of her and various parts of her body. The doctors would come in by the room-full. They would nod politely and leave, whispering about us out in the hall. Somehow that was a sign of respect for our privacy, but it felt more like children telling secrets. When I got tired of their chatter I would walk out into their midst, and they would disperse, leaving with little eye contact. It seemed like a victory when they left, but instead they were replaced with the sight of all the other children who were ill. Some seemed fine despite their conditions. Others were bald, gray and listless. Which fate awaits us?

Entering the Maze

"I'm sorry, but your child has cancer." To hear these words from a doctor is every parent's worst nightmare. And yet this bad news is passed on to thousands of parents each year. The incidence of cancer and other serious childhood illness is on the rise. More and more families are being forced to deal with the fact they are in the midst of a disturbing trend. Our children are increasingly facing terminal illness.

The road through such illness is unpaved and uncharted for most of us. Few parents have dealt with more than a few standard bouts of chicken pox, stomachaches or perhaps a trip to the emergency room for stitches before being forced on this confusing and strenuous journey. We are completely unprepared to manage the emotional stress, financial burden, time commitments and drudgery of helping our children through their ailments.

In *A Window to Heaven*, Dr. Diane M. Komp compares the trials parents face with a seriously ill child to those of Abraham and Sarah from the Bible, when Abraham was commanded by the Lord to climb a mountain in the land of Moriah to sacrifice his son, Isaac. As Dr. Komp puts it:

> Moriah is not only treacherous but ugly. A few hundred yards ahead I see the bare reminder of the trail that was last pursued to the top. I have never seen undergrowth spring back as fast as on Moriah, making it more difficult for newcomers to find the previously blazed trail. The vegetation on Moriah seems to have germinated in Hades, implanting itself as mature brush when the winds blow it in. The thorn bushes here do not even bother with the mockery of berries. No one who comes here would be fooled anyway, and none can escape the nasty encounter by choosing an easier path.[1]

The trials of Moriah leave our spirits bloodied and broken, seemingly unable to care for ourselves, let alone our children. Yet our little ones will look to us from the very start to provide them with the support they need to get through the most challenging experience they will face in their lifetime. Most of us will doubt our ability to provide that support on an ongoing basis. At times the situation seems too much, and we crumble under the pressure. But then moments come when we feel impervious to the pain, almost numb and cold in relation to the outside world. We ride an emotional roller coaster that goes through a seemingly endless cycle of ups and downs. In the end, our ability to manage those ups and downs is what helps us remain sane in an insane situation.

But as you enter the maze of childhood illness, your emotions seem anything but manageable. In her book *On Death and Dying*[2], Dr. Elisabeth Kubler-Ross details the various stages people go through in dealing with terminal illness. Although Dr. Ross' message is intended to describe how adult patients feel about their impending death, these stages are applicable to the parents of seriously ill children. Perhaps by understanding the cycles of our emotions, we can gain a better perspective on how to deal with them, while also learning how to best care for all the new and special needs of our kids.

The cycle starts with our reaction to the news of serious illness and ends with our ultimate ability (or lack of it) to deal with it. If I were to extrapolate Dr. Ross' findings to our children's situation, the typical parent might go through the following five stages:

1. After a brief period of shock upon first hearing the news, we enter the first stage—denial. This is rarely total denial, but more often a delay in our willingness to deal with what we've just heard. This stage can last minutes or months.

2. Once denial is no longer possible, we move into the second stage—anger. We often become bitter toward and frustrated by almost anything or anyone around us, especially those with more normal circumstances. We wonder why the illness has "chosen" to invade our lives rather than someone else's.

3. The third stage is bargaining. We negotiate with doctors or God for more time or better circumstances. When we realize this is not possible, we may slip back into anger or denial.

4. The fourth stage is depression. Here the anger and manipulation turn into despair. Because we know nothing can be done, a sense of hopelessness invades every aspect of our being. We do not deal with the illness; we just feel sad about it.

5. The final state is acceptance, when we acknowledge the illness and deal with it in a more constructive manner, often with a sense of hope something will happen to turn around our situation. This is *not* a kind of hope that leads to denial, but rather a realization that "it's not over until it's over."

And it is the hope to which we must all cling. Otherwise, we are left with hopelessness. For me, this hopelessness was what led me to slip into depression. It's also what made moving into acceptance hard for me. But we *must* ultimately move on to acceptance, if only for a brief period of time. I say this because most people go through these cycles more often than once. I went through each one of the five stages every time Amanda had a setback. The trick is to move through the process as quickly as possible to reach *hopeful* acceptance, the place where we can try to do something positive about our situation, no matter how devastating it might be. Only then can we begin to cultivate some sense of control, peace and hope.

Finding hope and acceptance is a critical part of the journey for both you and your child. Until you deal with your own emotions and attitude toward your child's illness, you will not be able to provide the physical and psychological support he or she needs so desperately. Furthermore, your decision making will be irrational. Your emotional state will rub off on your child, spouse, friends and family, ultimately making them as insecure and as angry as you are.

None of the five stages is bad. In fact, moving through each of them is healthy. If you get stuck in denial, anger or depression, however, you will never find peace and neither will your child. Seek help if you feel trapped. Otherwise, merely take note of how you're feeling and recognize it for what it is—a natural response to a difficult situation. In time, you'll find a way to deal with it.

Remember your circumstances will take you to places you don't want to be, but they cannot dictate how you feel once you get there. Seek the place inside of you where you can go to find peace, and then teach your child to access that part of him- or herself. Your child needs a safe and joyful refuge. You can give that to him or her more often than you think.

---

1. Taken from *A Window to Heaven* by Diane Komp, M.D Copyright © 1992 by Diane Komp. Used by permission of Zondervan Publishing House.

2. Adapted with the permission of Simon & Schuster from *On Death and Dying* by Elisabeth Kubler-Ross. Copyright © 1969 by Elisabeth Kubler-Ross.

CHAPTER 2

The First Weeks—Keeping Up With the System

"We cannot tell what may happen to us in the strange medley of life. But we can decide what happens in us—how we can take it, what we do with it—and that is what really counts in the end. How to take the raw stuff of life and make it a thing of worth and beauty—that is the test of living."

—Joseph Fort Newton

A Letter to Amanda: June 1991

Dear Amanda,

Today is the beginning of the beginning. Just one week ago they told us your condition was worse than expected. Your liver is involved along with your ears and skin, which means your disease is spreading throughout your body. The "wait and see" approach won't work here. They need to treat you very aggressively.

As I sit here looking at you, you are asleep. One hour ago, you came out of surgery, and now they are pumping chemotherapy into your veins through a catheter they have implanted under your skin. It goes directly into your heart to

13

*move the medicine through your body quickly. It's all hap-
pened so fast. You're just a child. How can this be?*

*Your mother and I watched you being wheeled into surgery
with your pink, stuffed bunny still in your hands. You were
sound asleep from the medication, which gave us some peace.
At least you weren't afraid anymore. This past week had
been horrible. They put you through tests almost every day.
Your little body was dwarfed by the machines they used on
you. We had to hold you down or restrain you forcibly through
it all. You are very angry at us right now. You want us to
save you, but we cannot. I cannot. I feel so helpless. I feel like
a failure. Daddies are supposed to take care of their little
girls. I seem to have gotten this all wrong.*

Journal Entry: June 1991

*Not sure who or what will hurt her next, Amanda becomes
agitated each time someone walks into the room. Even the
hourly blood pressure check has become very stressful. She
trusts no one, especially Deborah or me. Torture from strangers she can rationalize. But pain from her parents is too
outrageous to comprehend.*

*During her last temperature check, she grew inpatient and
would not allow it any longer. Since she was running a fever,
the nurse persisted, and I once again found myself holding
her down. At first she fought against me violently, seemingly
searching for some control in a desperate situation. Her face
turned purple, her mouth shut tight, and her back arched in
resistance for several minutes. But then, in the midst of the
struggle, she gave up. Her body went limp, she closed her
eyes and let out her breath, making a sound I will never
forget. It was the sigh of a broken spirit.*

*Minutes later, after the nurse had left, we watched her lie
down on the bed and close her eyes. She was not asleep, but
lay still as though she was. There was no peace in this still-*

ness, only the sadness you feel minutes after you realize you've lost something significant. And then to punctuate the moment, her eyes opened and she began to speak. Her tone was no longer one of defiance, but of pleading. She searched our eyes, looking for the compassion she had remembered in us not so long ago. Her voice started soft, but grew in intensity as she continued. "I never do bad again," she said. "Please no more 'owies,' and I never do bad again. PLEASE!"

Her words stopped, but her searching did not. Her eyes darted back and forth to Deborah and me, stopping only momentarily to see if she had connected with either one of us. Although our hearts were breaking, our response was quick and simultaneous. "Amanda, you're not being punished, honey. The doctors are trying to make you better."

Our attempts to console her continued, but she stopped listening long before we finished. She sensed immediately that our words would bring no change to her situation. Her head fell back to the pillow, and her eyes closed once again. She did not speak until the next morning.

Keeping Up With the System

The initial shock of the news about Amanda was quickly replaced with confusion as we began a wild ride into the health-care system. Three days after receiving the likely diagnosis from a local dermatologist, we were sent to a children's hospital in downtown Chicago for a series of tests to confirm the diagnosis. Five days and many tests later, Amanda underwent surgery and began chemotherapy.

I don't think I'd ever been through so much change in such a short period of time, nor will I ever again. All at once we were thrust into an onslaught of new experiences. Any one of these predicaments we encountered would be weighty by itself, but when slammed together into a few days, they were enough to push a normal person over the edge. For example, consider the following challenges that parents must face during the first sixty days of their experience:

- You are introduced to the complexities of acute hospital care, including a wide variety of specialists, most of whom you never knew existed. Medical terminology that sounds like Greek or Latin (because some of it is); and long hours of waiting while ten different hospital departments try to "fit you in" on their busy schedules become almost standards. The term "hurry up and wait" must have been coined by someone getting medical care in a hospital.

  At the same time, you enter the maze of insurance regulations, which have become stricter in this age of health-care reform. (This issue alone is complex enough to warrant an entire chapter. See Chapter 4.)

- You are introduced to your child's disease for the first time. If you're not a biology major, learning what you need to know can be like trying to learn a foreign language—but the stakes are higher. You need to learn as much as you can about the disease in one day because you will have to make decisions about your child's well-being based on your limited knowledge and restricted ability to communicate.

- You must become acutely sensitive to the immediate emotional needs of your child. Although you may have an intuitive sense for helping your child through difficult times, getting him or her through the trauma of acute care will test those intuitions.

- You must become an expert at time management. In our case, for example, the hospital is two hours away and Amanda's inpatient visits last anywhere from five to fourteen days. Her outpatient visits last six to twelve hours. But we also have another daughter to care for, a full-time job to maintain and a household to run. Routine activities such as grocery shopping and house cleaning are often left undone for weeks at a time.

- The financial burden of any hospital stay can be consuming. In an instant, you're faced with thousands of dollars of debt. You're lucky if you happen to have insurance, but that doesn't pay for everything. All insurance plans are different, but most policies cover only what is "reasonable," which is rarely what your medical bills actually turn out to be. You are responsible for the difference between these "reasonable" reimbursements and the actual bill, as well as all deductibles, co-payments and prescription services. You also incur thousands of dollars of additional expenses your insurance company never considers, such as day care for your other children, travel expenses to the hospital (with overnight expenses) and charges for additional services that you would normally perform yourself but now you just don't have the time.

- Stress levels reach an all-time high during these early weeks. You discover a whole set of emotions you never knew existed, exacerbated by sleeplessness because of worry or all-night care for your child. Attempting to deal with these emotions while remaining "in control" for your child, spouse, friends, family and co-workers puts you on a tightrope you have never had to walk before.

Looking back on the magnitude of change, I'm not sure how our family survived intact The burden seemed to overpower us so many times I can't count the number of breakdowns (large and small) our family went through, either together or separately. But a singular focus on getting your child through times of crisis is what pulls you through in the long run, especially during the first few weeks. Your complete focus on your child's care is required to keep priorities in line and bring some sense of clarity to a complex set of circumstances.

Even with that focus, a number of things can slip through the cracks as you blast through the first few weeks and months. You can minimize the amount of debris left behind, however. I offer the following suggestions to anyone going through the process for the first time:

1. Keep a detailed medical journal. Write down everything your doctor tells you, even if you think you will remember. Chances are you'll forget it later when something else seems more important. Also keep track of *all* medications. On several occasions my wife, Deborah, and I halted a nurse who was about to give Amanda the wrong medicine or the wrong amount. Nurses and doctors are human; they make mistakes.

2. Don't hesitate to ask any question, even if it seems stupid. Keep asking it until you understand the answer. You're not there to impress the doctors; you're there to find the best care for your child. Keep a piece of paper and a pen with you at all times to write down your questions as soon as you think of them, and then bring your list to each visit with the doctor. Your head is spinning during the first few months, and you'll routinely forget even the most important questions when you finally have the time to ask them.

3. Participate in your child's care. Understand what the doctors are doing and why they're doing it. Don't be afraid to stand up to your doctor if something doesn't feel right. Good doctors will appreciate your concern and will spend time with you to walk through the decision-making process. I'll talk more about this in the next chapter.

4. Get a second, third or fourth opinion. We went to three experts before moving forward on Amanda's liver transplant.

5. Once you've come to agree with your doctors, trust them. If you've checked out their credentials and the treatment

they've recommended, let them do their jobs. A time comes to let go and let the experts take over.

6. Find out everything you can about your child's illness. Many resources for information exist, even if your child has a rare disease.

7. Recognize you can't get *everything* done and let some things go. It's OK to be in chaos for a while. You have bigger things to worry about.

8. Find time for yourself. You can easily lose yourself in this early time but don't let it happen. *Your physical and mental well-being is in the best interest of your child.* Being a martyr or being completely selfless is a self-destructive path that will ultimately be destructive to your child. Take time to take care of yourself, even though that seems impossible.

This is certainly not a comprehensive list, but it contains some of the most critical points to get you through the first few months. The most important point to remember is you cannot control everything. Quickly identify where you can help and do everything you can in those few areas; but also learn when to let go and allow others to help you. You can't make it alone. Recognize that now, and you'll be a saner person for it.

If you have family, friends or neighbors, accept their help when they offer it. If not, seek out services that provide support to single caregivers. Ask a hospital social worker to guide you to the places where you can find help. Most hospitals also have created support groups for parents that meet regularly. Look to them for assistance. You'll be amazed at how many "strangers" want to pitch in to help you in your time of need.

For me, this was one of the hardest lessons to learn. I spent years trying to be strong and independent about Amanda's illness. I didn't want to bother anybody by talking about it, and I certainly didn't want to be a burden by asking for help. When we absolutely needed assistance, I felt guilty about asking for it and obligated to somehow return the favor. But the deeper we slipped into our situation, the more help we needed.

Perhaps that is one of the things I had to learn in this process—how to need other people, how to accept assistance without embarrassment and with thanks. Maybe God was trying to show me I need other people, no matter how independent I want to be. No one can make it on his or her own, whatever the circumstances. Receiving and giving are all part of the same energy of His love. The sooner we realize that, the sooner we will be blessed by the lives of those around us; and they, in turn, can be blessed by our lives too.

———————————

CHAPTER 3

Working With the Medical Staff

"Although a physician, I am only human . . . parents and doctors alike, we must seek someone worthy of our trust, especially when the future is uncertain."

—Diane M. Komp, M.D.

Journal Entry: January 1, 1994

Happy New Year? According to whom? It's 2 A.M. and Amanda's IV is shot again. This is the third IV since Christmas. I hate IVs. They've tried four times to start another one, but they keep blowing out her veins. Amanda is hysterical. All she wants to do is sleep, but she won't go down until the IV is in. I won't let anyone else try to start one until an expert arrives. In the last week we've had no fewer than twelve attempts to get three good IVs started. We've been waiting two hours now for an anesthesiologist, but they're all out celebrating the advent of a new year. The nurses are getting impatient because Amanda is four hours late with her medications. They want to try again, but I'm holding firm on this one.

Journal Entry: May 1995

It had been forty-five minutes since we handed him the CT scan. Why was he taking so long? It couldn't be good news if

21

it was taking this long. But it had to be good news. She'd been looking too good recently. I wouldn't accept anything but good news.

Finally, he emerged from behind the door. His look of intensity contrasted to his normal calm. He walked quickly toward the play area where all the families wait with their children. And when he approached us, he didn't have to say a word. We've been down this road before. We know the gestures; we can interpret the body language. "It's back, and it doesn't look good," he said.

And with that, the parents around us went silent. They stared at us to see our reaction, but then realized how uncomfortable the situation was. Their eyes turned away, but their ears were still perked to hear our conversation. No one spoke except the children, who played on without a clue. Amanda was still focused on her toy of choice.

With the relative silence, he realized that he should have pulled us away from the crowd before making the announcement. "We're going to radiology to get an ultrasound right now," he said in an effort to bring closure for the group around us. But it was too late. They were part of the moment now. So when our backs turned as we headed out the door, their eyes returned to our family drama. I stopped momentarily, and with Amanda in my arms, I looked back to where they were sitting. Each of the fathers turned away immediately, but the mothers looked on just long enough to share their concern.

Once out of the area, I quickly moved into the mode of gathering information. How bad was it? Where was it? What tests were we going to do? Who did we have to see? (I'm amazingly rational during the early stages of getting the news. It's only after the initial frenzy that I fall apart.) He responded quickly, almost in a rushed, abrupt fashion. He was even walking quickly. It was hard to keep up with him, both in pace and conversation.

When we got to radiology, he told us to wait. He disappeared into another room to talk to some other doctors for about five minutes while we sat silently with Amanda. When he emerged, he took a deep breath and gave us eye contact for the first time since walking into the play area. He gave us the plan of action and then began to walk away. But he stopped himself and turned back to Amanda. His hand came down around her face, and he squatted to be at her level. And then he said to her in a very soft tone, "You're a beautiful child, Amanda MacLellan."

As he spoke those words, his eyes glistened just a little more than they had one second earlier. "Yeah, I am," came Amanda's reply. And with that we all smiled, with some half-hearted laughter thrown in for extra effort. A few moments of silence passed, and then he turned and walked down the long hallway. I noticed his pace was slower and his head was down, shaking in disbelief. This man is grieving too.

Journal Entry: September 1995

It's 1 A.M., and I'm staying with Amanda in the hospital tonight. After six days of not sleeping much at all, I was finally able to drift off around midnight. But at 12:30, the senior resident in charge for the night came into our room and called me out into the hall to discuss a concern about Amanda. Since her condition had stabilized about 24 hours ago and this was not one of her doctors, I was a little confused as to what this was all about.

As I stumbled out the door, still unable to open my eyes from the deep sleep I had just entered, this young doctor immediately launched into a lecture about how it was not my place to make decisions about Amanda's care. As I slowly came around, I realized he was talking about my request of a nurse earlier that evening to let Amanda sleep rather than wake her up to take her blood pressure and temperature. She had been wakened four times during the previous hour for various reasons, and I wanted her to rest. Sleep has always been her greatest healing mechanism, and I could tell from my touch that she had no significant fever. I've gotten to the point where I'm accurate to within two-tenths of a degree.

Still, it seemed important to him, so I explored it further, though by now I was pretty pissed off at his attitude, and I was becoming rather testy myself. As it turned out, he was not that concerned about Amanda's temperature, but wanted his efforts documented in the records so that neither he nor the hospital would be liable in the event of a problem. He further stated that Amanda was not my responsibility and that I should "leave it to the experts."

Amanda is not my responsibility? And this man who read her chart for the first time some twenty minutes ago knows more about her condition than I do? I don't think so. "I'm her father," I said. "She is my primary responsibility. It seems you're more concerned about legal liabilities than you are about my daughter." And with that he stuttered into threats of calling her oncologist so that he would not be accountable if problems occurred.

So out of respect for her oncologist, who relies as much on art, listening and watching as he does on science, I let the resident take Amanda's vital signs. As expected, everything was fine. But now Amanda is agitated, and I'm wide awake. It looks like I'll be moving on to day seven without much sleep. But at least some resident is walking the halls feeling better protected from the legal system.

Working With the Medical Staff

Somewhere in the middle of my writing Chapter 2, Amanda began having daily migraines and fevers over 103 degrees. We began to track her condition very closely because any child on chemotherapy who develops a fever over 101 degrees needs to be taken to the emergency room immediately. But after four years of dragging Amanda to the ER as many as two or three times a week, we've learned to wait things out awhile. We've been scolded severely by several doctors for not bringing her right in, but these emergencies are very stressful on Amanda. Each trip to the ER involves pulling her out of bed in the middle of the night (when she always seems to experience the fevers), driving two hours to the hospital for a rush of activity including taking blood, starting an IV (a very painful process for any child) and an all-night session of test after test after test. Frequently, we'd end up in the hospital for a two-week course of IV antibiotics "just to be safe." More often than not, the doctors never identified the source of her original fever and sent us home without any answers.

After about a year of this drill, Deborah and I realized Amanda tends to spike fevers for no apparent reason. The trips to the ER were torture, and the stress seemed to make her more susceptible to other, more dangerous infections. But a child on chemo can get extremely ill, even close to death, very quickly. We've seen Amanda go from completely normal to very, very sick within an hour. As a consequence, we've had to walk a fine line between being overly cautious and somewhat reckless in a critical situation. That line has often put us at odds with the medical staffs of several hospitals, but it is one we felt was critical for Amanda's quality of life and well-being.

Finding the balance between playing by the rules of medicine and protecting your child from a sometimes overly aggressive and insensitive health-care system is what this chapter is all about. Discovering middle ground is not easy and will differ for each family, each hospital and each doctor. I'll share with you our perspective that has evolved and been reinforced by our personal experience over the last five years.

Challenging the System

As Deborah and I first began to feel bringing Amanda to the hospital was sometimes hurting her more than helping her, we'd ask questions to get an opinion from the doctors. As you might imagine, we got a wide variety of responses. Some listened very well, while others blew us off completely. No matter how kind or rude they were, all of them ultimately insisted we needed to bring her in each and every time—and we did for at least another six months.

During those six months, our questions turned into direct challenges to the decisions being made, which in turn led to our insistence that a better way to handle her care be found. As we grew more persistent, we found we still drew a wide variety of responses from the medical community. Some doctors continued to listen, but then respectfully disagreed with our opinion. Many became increasingly annoyed with our questions, however, and began to imply or state directly we were out of our league and should back off. It was during this time we discovered numerous obstacles to finding real balance for a child caught up in the "system," including:

- Doctors who don't believe you should participate in your child's care

- Doctors who do everything by the book, no matter what the circumstances maybe with your child

- Multiple doctors with different opinions

- Multiple doctors with the same opinion, who all disagree with what you think is best for your child

- Information overload

- Doctors who are more worried about being sued than about doing what's right

- A health-care system that is very complex and confusing

- Your own lack of knowledge and expertise on what's best for your child

These obstacles often connect in different ways to make it very difficult to determine how to provide the best care for your child. In the end, I believe it boils down to a difference of opinion as to what "best care" really means. Your doctors probably define it as the best possible science, combined with a well-defined health-care system. As parents, Deborah and I define it as quality of life, in combination with the best available scientific medical treatment.

In order to understand how those different perspectives are reached, you need to understand how our health-care system works—and how that system tends to overwhelm the families who are forced to deal with it.

How the System Works

The health-care system starts with something called *primary care*. As the word primary would indicate, this is the first line of medicine; it's your local doctor, pediatrician or clinic setting. It's where you go when you have the flu or some other ailment that needs attention but is not life threatening. Typically, this is the doctor who notices something is not right and sends you to a specialist for further examination. If the specialist finds something wrong, you may move on to the next level—acute care.

Acute care is the level used to describe a hospital setting. Hospitals typically fall into one of three different categories: local community hospitals that handle mostly routine procedures, specialty hospitals that focus on very specific treatments such as cancer, and major medical centers that handle the most complex cases. Major medical centers are often called referral hospitals because other acute care institutions refer their most difficult problems to them.

Some of these same centers are also called teaching hospitals because they are associated with medical schools. As the name implies, medical students and recent medical school graduates are taught how to be doctors by working with more experienced physicians. Many children's hospitals and major medical centers are associated with medical schools, so you will most likely see these new doctors care for your child on a fairly regular basis. For that reason you need to know more about them. Like the military, teaching hospitals have a regimented hierarchy of rank, privilege and (hopefully) skill as students and doctors advance through the system.

- *Medical Students* are people who have decided they want to be doctors and are attending medical school. Med students don't usually show up in the hospitals until they are almost done with school and even then they have little contact with patients.

- *Interns* have just graduated from medical school and are now officially called medical doctors (MDs). On more than one occasion, Amanda has been an intern's very first patient— first patient ever. Twice I have watched an intern go ask another doctor how to write a prescription properly. (If that doesn't inspire confidence, I don't know what will!)

- *Residents* are doctors who made it through internship and are now studying a specialty. The interns report through older residents, who also may have rank distinctions such second-year resident and senior resident.

- *Attending Physicians* are "real" doctors who are in charge of the residents. Residents will often consult with the "attending" to make sure they all have followed proper procedure.

- *Specialists* are doctors who have chosen to focus on a particular medical specialty. Specialists have made it through all the rigors of the system and teach residents to become more proficient in their specific specialty. It's a kind of apprentice program.

The bottom line is you will encounter lots of different kinds of doctors with different skill levels when you go into the hospital. When Amanda gets admitted, she's often first examined by an intern. If the intern is concerned about Amanda's condition he or she will call a resident. If that resident is concerned, the call then goes to a senior resident, who might call the attending to see her, who might call Amanda's oncologist, who might send an apprentice, who might then send for a different specialist.

In the first few trips to the hospital, I was totally confused by this parade of doctors. I didn't know who was responsible for Amanda's care or why so many people kept coming in to examine her. I asked questions of brand-new doctors who were not experienced enough to answer my questions, which made me fear she was getting substandard care, which made me get defensive, which made working with the medical staff difficult. This was all compounded by the fact Amanda was being seen by several departments within a hospital, and each had its own unique layers of doctors. I saw a Doonesbury once that summed up all of this very nicely.

Doonesbury

BY GARRY TRUDEAU

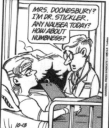 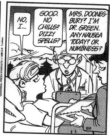 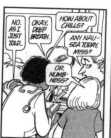 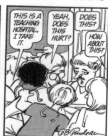

It's perplexing, to say the least. I am still sometimes confused by the doctors who show up in Amanda's room to examine her. But over time, you become used to having a vast number of people involved in your case. You learn whom to ask what questions, whom to seek out and whom to avoid. In effect, you learn to work the system instead of having it work you. You begin to learn you do have a say in what happens to your son or daughter and you can and should participate in your child's care. Although most doctors are caring, sensitive, knowledgeable people, not all of them take into account the total impact their decisions have on your child. Even the best doctors make mistakes or disagree with each other on the best course of action for your child.

Working the System

So what do you do? How do you work through all the different opinions, perspectives, styles and recommendations? I offer the following advice based on our experience.

Rule #1: Find out who is in charge of your child's care.

There will always be one doctor who is ultimately responsible for your child. This person is sometimes called the primary physician. Your primary physician may be your pediatrician, but most likely will be a specialist. In Amanda's case, the oncologist is her primary physician. Although doctors from several other departments participate in her care, they are called into her case by her oncologist. The specialist, in effect, calls in other specialists.

For example, one week Deborah and I ultimately decided to take Amanda to the hospital. Her fevers topped 105 degrees for three straight days, then she broke out in a rash. Her oncologist called in the liver transplant team, infectious disease physicians and dermatologists. Each of these specialists reported his or her opinions back to the oncologist, who made the final decision as to Amanda's treatment. After five days of antibiotics, they couldn't identify the source of the fevers and sent her home. Sound familiar? In this case, however, the antibiotics severely aggravated her kidneys, causing more problems for Amanda than when we took her in. This is another reason we tend to avoid "preventative" treatment.

Rule #2: When in doubt, always default in favor of what your primary physician is telling you.

If doctors express conflicting opinions about what is best for your child, do what your primary physician recommends. He or she probably knows your child's case best and is the most knowledgeable about what has worked well and what hasn't. They also have the most information about what's happening at each particular stage of a hospital admission, and complete continuum of care.

Rule #3: When in doubt, always default to what any doctor is telling you.

Although we often challenge Amanda's doctors about their treatment plan, we usually end up doing exactly what they want us to do, even if we're not sure it makes sense. Most doctors are very capable and know far more about medicine than you or I. In the vast majority of cases, they have the best interest of your child at heart. If you have any doubt about a decision, default in favor of the doctors.

Rule #4: Beware of defensive medicine.

If something feels excessive, your doctor may be practicing defensive medicine. In my experience, defensive medicine comes in two types: legal and just-in-case. The legal type is when doctors do something merely because they're afraid of being sued if they don't. Unfortunately, litigation-happy America has forced doctors to take the legal system into account in almost every decision they make.

For instance, if chances are only one in a thousand your child has a particular problem, logic would tell you that you probably don't need to test for it. The legal system, however, might penalize your doctor severely if that one-in-a-thousand

chance came true. As such, many doctors will run several potentially very painful tests just to make sure that they are "covered"
if taken to court. Your child is the one who suffers as a result.

Just-in-case defensive medicine is practiced by the overly
cautious doctor who wants to test for the one-in-a-million disease just in case it's the source of the problem. This is particularly
true with newer doctors who don't have enough experience to
rule out certain problems just by observing the situation. They're
also incredibly concerned about doing the wrong thing (for all the
right reasons), so they'll do much more than is required. Again,
your child is the one who suffers the pain or aggravation of the
testing, while you bear the burden of the expense of the procedures and the anguish of watching your child go through them.

As you gain more experience with your child, you may
also find this is true in more routine, "reasonable" testing procedures. For example, every time Amanda came into the ER with
a high fever, the doctors ordered a spinal tap to check for men-
ingitis, which is fairly common among kids on chemotherapy. A
spinal tap is a very painful procedure, incredibly traumatic for
anybody but especially for a child. They would justify the test
based on her fever and irritability—standard stuff for any doctor. If they mentioned the case in the doctors' lounge, they'd all
nod their heads it was the right thing to do.

But as her parents, we know how Amanda behaves every
time she comes to the ER. She is naturally irritable because she
knows what's coming and is angry about it. She's fed up with
being sick all the time and is upset she has been pulled out of
bed to run the drill yet one more time. We also know she runs
fevers routinely and her temperature hits 103 degrees fairly regularly. Consequentially, after several spinal taps, we began refusing
the procedure to allow doctors more time to observe her before
making a final decision on the test.

The first time I refused the tap within ten minutes I had
three doctors, each with increasing authority, come to the small
ER exam room to tell me what a terrible mistake I was making.

I persisted, however, and Amanda turned out to have a very common virus. I've probably refused five spinal taps since then, and I get a somewhat similar response from the doctors each time. Now I'm just a little more confident in my choice. You need, however, to consider two critical points when making these types of decisions. First, never be smug. Although I'm now more certain about when to step in and refuse a test, I always take into account the potentially serious downside if I'm wrong. I track Amanda's condition very aggressively and report any changes I witness to the doctors.

Second, refusing a test once does not mean you refuse it every time. Sometimes when we've gone to the ER we allowed the tap immediately. If Amanda seems particularly ill, I feel too far outside my comfort zone to refuse the test. Remember, when in doubt, always do what the doctor recommends.

Rule #5: Pain is inevitable.

I considered refusing a test many times merely because I didn't want to put Amanda through it, or because she pleaded with me not to have it performed. As a parent, you can't allow those considerations to cloud your judgment. You must do what's right, even if it means your child will experience pain.

Just this past summer Amanda was diagnosed with lymphoma for the second time. We learned of the diagnosis less than a day after her surgery and only hours after discovering how extensive the cancer was throughout her body. We weren't at all convinced she was going to live, and we debated whether to treat her or take her home to die.

Her bladder was extended because she had not urinated for almost twenty-four hours, and the nurse told me Amanda would have to be catheterized. (The lingering effects of the anesthesia were blocking her ability to push out the urine.) Amanda dislikes this procedure intensely and promised she would pee if we just gave her more time. The nurse gave us fifteen minutes to make it happen or she would have to insert the catheter. Two hours later, we still had no luck. I had been holding Amanda up on the bedpan for almost the entire time, while appealing to the nurse to give her yet another chance. Finally, I had to tell Amanda it was time. She screamed and pleaded with me not to call the nurse, but I had to. It was becoming a dangerous situation, and her bladder might burst.

It took the nurse twenty minutes to insert the catheter. During that time, Amanda took out her rage on me, screaming, "I hate you, Daddy, I hate you. You're making them do this to me. Why are you doing this? I hate you, Daddy, I hate you." Eventually, I collapsed against the wall and fell to the floor. I wasn't sure if she would live through the night. Would these be her last words to me? Would these be her last thoughts of my love?

I wanted to push the nurses aside and rush her out of the room. I wanted to save her, if only once. I wanted her to see how much pain I was in too—that it mattered to me she was hurting. I wanted to end the misery. But I could not. Nor could I stop the hundreds of times when the pain was a lot more unbearable than a "mere" catheter insertion. Ultimately, as parents we have to recognize that our children must go through some of these trials in order to be made well. And they just may blame us for all of it.

Rule #6: Confusion is inevitable.

Sooner or later, you'll get conflicting reports from all the different doctors involved in your case, or your primary contact will change his or her mind midstream in a treatment plan. Sometimes these contradictions or changes in direction can be very confusing and disheartening. Just when you think you understand what's going on and have mentally adjusted to a particular course of action, some doctor says something to weaken your confidence in the current plan, or your primary physician suddenly supports a path completely different from the one he or she recommended just a day earlier.

You have a choice here, which can reduce the confusion. You can ask your doctor not to share anything with you that is speculative or not yet fully supported by research. Your doctor will tell you only what he or she *knows* and will keep the rest to him- or herself. While changes in direction should still be expected, the amount of confusion will be greatly reduced.

The problem with this option is you may have to wait a long time to get answers to the hundreds of questions running through your mind. Some tests are not definitive for several days, and even then the doctors may require several more days to gather enough data to determine a course of action. In the meantime, you're left wondering what's happening and may not be getting some potentially good news along the way.

Deborah and I have always chosen to get each piece of information as soon as it becomes available. But while we are always very well informed, we also get caught up in conflicting test results, different opinions from doctors, miscommunication on next steps and a wide variety of other contradictions that put our emotions on a roller coaster of extreme highs and deep lows. It isn't easy, and you must prepare yourself for bad news if you want as much news as possible on what's happening around you.

Rule #7: *Aggravation is cumulative.*

Each doctor involved in your child's case will call for a series of tests to help diagnose a problem in a particular specialty. Remember, any one of these doctors could be practicing defensive medicine or may be just particularly thorough in approach. Although most of these tests seem harmless to each doctor, the cumulative effect on you and your child can be overwhelming.

Even if you have only three doctors involved in a case and each calls for only three tests on a particular day, that's nine tests. You also have to take into account the nurse is coming in every hour or so to take vital signs, draw blood or do a cursory examination. In addition, a parade of interns comes into the room to examine your child for the benefit of their learning, not of your child's care, and the specialists come in to examine your child as well.

Now consider that your son or daughter doesn't feel good, is filled with medicine that may affect behavior and may have been forced to eat. Mix it all together and you've got an incredibly stressful situation. There were days when Amanda went through very painful procedures without complaining, only to freak out when the nurse wanted to take her temperature.

The cumulative effect of the constant poking and prodding is stressful for everyone concerned. Your doctor, however, may not have knowledge of (or appreciation for) the many procedures being performed on your child. When you challenge a test or procedure that seems completely routine and simple, the doctor may think you're being an unreasonable, overprotective parent.

For instance, Amanda gets several CT scans a year. (You may know them as CAT scans, which are a series of X-rays that form a somewhat three-dimensional view of the body.) CT scans are fairly commonplace in modern medicine and seem like a simple test to your average physician. To Amanda, however, the scan is not so simple. Each time a CT is ordered, she has to get an IV, which can take as long as two hours of very painful needle sticks before one is working. Next, she has to drink a large amount of a contrast chemical to help her organs show up better on the X-ray. This contrast liquid makes her feel very sick. She also has to lie perfectly still on a table for about a half hour in a very uncomfortable position, in a room that is kept very cold so that the computers involved in the CT machine don't overheat. She also has to be injected through her IV with another contrast material that burns terribly as it goes through the body.

Add to the CT scan the other eight tests for the day, and you can begin to see how the "simple" testing is not so simple and how the stress builds. Aggravation is cumulative, but your doctor may not see it that way. You are the only one who has the total picture, and it's your job to make sure your doctors understand what that looks like, whether they want to see it or not.

Rule #8: Spirit is just as important as body.

Perhaps one of the greatest failings of most physicians is their complete reliance on science. They often fail to recognize that by reducing stress, by increasing love and by trusting intuition, we can often heal more quickly than with drugs and surgical procedures. Our spirits have an amazing capacity to heal our bodies when given the chance. But that takes time, faith and trust in something less tangible than scientific method or a medical book.

Many times we knew what Amanda needed was not another test, but a chance to get out of the hospital—a chance to sleep in her own bed without disruption. A chance to be with her sister, in familiar surroundings without the threat of another examination or needle prick. She often healed quickest at home.

Many doctors don't have that perspective because it's not in their training, nor would it hold up in a court of law if challenged. They will struggle with your attempts to provide such an environment and often make you feel as though you're doing something wrong. But I firmly believe safe, loving, positive surroundings are as important—if not more so—as science.

Summary

The *vast majority* of doctors are very good people who care a lot about their profession and their patients. Our family has been blessed with many, many doctors who are both very capable and very compassionate; men and women who take the time to listen not only to us, but to Amanda as well.

Some of Amanda's doctors have gone far above and beyond the call of duty to care for her needs. Amanda's liver doctor spent three hours in traffic driving to our house after he discovered her first cancerous tumor in a chest X-ray. We had left the hospital before he was shown the film, and he was so concerned about her immediate well-being he didn't want to wait to track us down on the phone.

In another instance, Amanda's cardiac surgeon and a hospital administrator spent four hours sorting through soiled linens looking for her favorite stuffed, pink bunny, which had been lost during her second heart surgery. (They never did find it.)

Many doctors are in the profession for both the love of medicine and their patients. But we've also discovered even the most capable and compassionate doctors are human beings just like you and me. They make mistakes and sometimes act more in their own best interests than in yours. Even so, you should *never* go against the advice of your doctor unless you feel absolutely certain you have more information than he or she does.

If you feel strongly about something that contrasts with your doctor's opinion, remember no one knows your child better than you do. Good doctors will recognize that and want your input. *The relationship you have with your doctor does not have to be adversarial* . Talk with your doctors. Make sure they understand your perspective and have all the information needed to make good decisions.

You are an important resource in determining the best next steps. Ask challenging questions about treatment plans to make sure you are completely comfortable. Without offending the doctor, your questions may stimulate new ideas that could lead to a better treatment plan.

In the process, give spirit a chance. Whether you consider it to be a force of God or merely the fighting will of a child is not important. Recognize that a loving, supportive, nourishing, safe environment can be just as important as the latest drug. You may find getting anyone to consider spirit in conjunction with body is a formidable task—but I urge you to accept the challenge.

---

1. Taken from *A Child Shall Lead Them* by Diane M. Komp, M.D. Copyright © 1993 by Diane M. Komp, M.D. Used by permission of Zondervan Publishing House. p. 132.

2. DOONESBURY © 1995 G.B. Trudeau. Reprinted with permission of UNIVERSAL PRESS SYNDICATE. All rights reserved.

CHAPTER 4

Managed Care—Living With Health-Care Reform

"A major fear consumers voice about Managed Care is that they will become seriously ill and the plan will not come through with the very best doctor or hospital. Finding a place to trust with your health is still largely up to you."

—U.S. News & World Report[1]

Journal Entry: September 1991

I can't stand it anymore. I spend hours on the phone trying to work through problems with the hundreds of bills that have piled up over the last four months. The insurance company tells me to call the hospital, and the hospital tells me to call the insurance company. I must spend about twenty hours a week sorting through all this stuff. It feels like I'm never going to get out of this trap.

Most of the bills are past due now, and I'm starting to get threatening letters from collection agencies. I don't think we're going to survive this financially. I thought I had a good insurance plan.

Journal Entry: July 1993

The insurance company has been calling all of Amanda's

doctors. They seem to be asking leading questions about the liver transplant which would indicate that they may not cover it. When I called to confront them, no one would answer my questions; but after about the tenth call, I finally got somebody to tell me that they weren't sure that the transplant "was in Amanda's best interest."

She'll die a slow and painful death within the next six months without a new liver. How can that be a better option?

Journal Entry: August 1993

The good news is that they finally approved the liver transplant. The bad news is that they're sending us to a different hospital—a hospital without a successful record in pediatric transplantation. We have the single best hospital in the world for pediatric liver transplants right here in Chicago and we can't go there.

Health-Care Reform and Managed Care

Imagine your doctor tells you the hospital can do nothing more for your daughter. She needs a new liver, and the hospital doesn't have a liver transplant program. Fortunately, however, the best pediatric liver transplant team in the country is only ten miles away.

Although the liver transplant sounds very scary, at least you happen to live near one of the best hospitals in the world for that procedure. Perhaps the best news of all is this particular hospital has pioneered what they call the "living related donor" liver transplant program. This allows a living family member to donate part of his or her liver (if it's a match), rather than wait for a cadaver liver.

By taking a piece of a relative's liver, the child's chances for recovery are vastly improved for several reasons. First, the liver is never frozen. It is taken directly from the donor and placed into the recipient, thus reducing damage to the organ. Second, the living related donor liver may be a better match for your child, which reduces the chance of rejection. Third, the donor liver is available for immediate transplantation. This allows a child to go into surgery before he or she becomes critically ill (which is often a necessary condition to get to the top of the organ waiting list). The healthier a child is going into surgery, the better the chances for recovery. And finally, an organ is virtually guaranteed for your child once a match has been made. Many children die while waiting for a cadaver liver.

Needless to say, you're very pleased to have such an opportunity for your child. Your hope and excitement build. But then your realize with all the commotion, you forgot to call your insurance company. Your employer just switched to a "managed care" plan, and you're supposed to call to get approval before going to a new hospital. So you dutifully make the call, expecting to fulfill your obligations and move on.

The woman on the other end of the phone informs you that you can't go to this "best chance" hospital because it's not in your employer's network of approved hospitals. If your daughter needs a liver transplant, she'll have to go to another hospital in Chicago —one that's not as experienced in pediatric liver transplants and does not offer the living donor program. In effect, you will be forced to watch your daughter slowly deteriorate until she is placed in the ICU during the last weeks of her life. Maybe, just maybe, an organ will become available in time.

But that's not all. As you muddle through the waiting period, one of your doctors calls to give you some disturbing news. Apparently, your insurance company has been calling around asking a lot of questions about your daughter's condition. In your doctor's opinion, the insurance company is trying to prove the liver transplant won't help your daughter's long-term prognosis and maybe they shouldn't "bother." So you call your insurance company and try to get some answers. Finally, someone admits the company is thinking about not covering the transplant. The words this person uses are, "We're not sure if it's in her best interest." Somehow you don't feel the company has her best interest at heart.

Obviously, this is our story. We spent months working it all out—many discouraging phone calls, letters and meetings. But we finally did it. We finally got her transplant approved at the hospital that offered the living donor program. After going through a series of tests, I was given the gift of serving as Amanda's liver donor, and today a little piece of me lives inside of her. We were the fiftieth living related liver donor pair at the hospital that introduced the procedure to the world. It was an awesome experience.

But the battle that was fought to give Amanda her best chance at life was completely draining. Even after getting the procedure approved, we spent two and a half years buried in paperwork created when we first stepped out of my employer's insurance network. And when I finally saw the light at the end of the paperwork tunnel, my company sold the division I worked for and I had to start the process all over again with a new employer using a new insurance company.

As anyone who's been in the hospital knows, dealing with insurance companies can be very difficult, if not impossible. Recent changes in our health-care system have created a whole new set of complexities that make health insurance coverage confusing at its best and seemingly evil at its worst. Still, those of us with insurance are the lucky ones. As we hear on the news almost every night, millions of Americans are without health insurance and desperate for some type of coverage. It's a difficult situation almost any way you look at it.

How did we get in this position? Why are so many without health-care insurance? And for those of us who have it, why is dealing with the companies that provide the coverage so difficult? Why does health-care insurance get more and more complex each year, while the coverage seems to offer less and less? And why were the Clintons unable to do anything about it?

I hope this chapter will answer some of those questions. I'll not even attempt to offer a solution for the current situation, but I will try to shed some light on it. Perhaps then you will understand what's happening when your insurance company or your hospital seems to offer a less than compassionate answer to some of your most important health coverage questions. In order to understand the present circumstances, I'll need to go back a few years and offer some perspective on where the problems started. Understanding where we've been makes understanding where we are today a lot easier.

A Quick History of the Health-Care System: It's Not the Money, It's the Money

As you might imagine, most of the issues center on money, specifically, how the care providers, hospitals, doctors, nursing homes, and so forth get paid for their services. In the 1960s and 1970s, these providers were paid under a "cost-plus" system, using the *cost* of a procedure *plus* a markup. Say you were playing softball and broke your finger trying to make a big play at home plate. Hospital A was right down the street, so you walked to the emergency room to get an X-ray. The ER staff confirmed your finger was broken, put it in a splint, taped it up and sent you home. The cost of fixing your broken finger at Hospital A was 100 dollars and the markup was 10 percent, so your insurance company was charged 110 dollars. The bill was paid.

But what if Hospital B was closer to your home, so you went to its ER instead of Hospital A? Hospital B handled your broken finger just as well as Hospital A would have, but it wasn't as cost-effective and the bill totaled 200 dollars. In this case, Hospital B charged your insurance company 220 dollars (200 dollars + 10 percent markup), and the bill was paid just as quickly as the bill for 110 dollars at Hospital A. As the consumer of the service, you weren't bothered a bit that it cost more at Hospital B than at Hospital A because your insurance company paid the bill. The increased cost didn't affect your payment.

Furthermore, what if Hospital C had the best reputation for emergency care, so you went out of your way to go there? The hospital just bought the best X-ray machine available, so it cost 300 dollars to diagnose and fix your broken finger. This hospital charged your insurance company 330 dollars, and the bill was paid just as quickly as it would have been at Hospital A or Hospital B. Once again, you didn't care about the increased cost because you didn't bear the financial burden. In fact, you didn't even know there was a difference in price among the three hospitals.

Think about the implications of a system that worked like this. Not only did the system not encourage cost efficiency, it actually rewarded providers that had higher costs. Consider our example with the broken finger for a minute. Did you notice Hospital A made only 10 dollars on the broken finger, while Hospital B made 20 dollars and Hospital C made 30 dollars, all for doing exactly the same thing? The most cost-effective hospital made the least profit. The inefficient hospital made a little bit more, and the big-spending hospital made the most amount of profit.

Not only did this system encourage higher costs at the provider level, it discouraged you from finding the best value care because the bill was paid no matter what choices you made. Although the profits made in our broken finger example don't seem too extreme, apply the same formulas to the cost of:

- Having a baby
- A triple heart bypass
- Cancer treatment
- Brain surgery
- Organ transplants

With this payment system in place, the costs for health-care services in America grew at a rapid rate. But hospitals loved it because they were making more and more money the higher the costs went. Doctors loved it because every test and procedure they ordered meant more money in the bank. We consumers didn't care because our employers paid our health insurance premiums, and the insurance companies paid the mounting health-care bills. All the while, we enjoyed the best health care in the world. In summary, this system was great for the *consumers* of health care (you and me) and the *providers* of health care (doctors and hospitals), but the *payors* of health care (those who actually paid the bills) were becoming concerned.

Among these payors of health care is our very own U. S. government, the single largest payor of health-care services in America. By 1980, the U.S. government was spending more than 9 percent of its total budget on health care, mostly on Medicare (government-paid health care for senior Americans) and Medicaid (government-paid health care for impoverished Americans). With the budget deficit widening and political pressure to reduce taxes increasing, the government had to do something about this out-of-control financial burden. In 1983 it introduced a new health-care payment scheme to replace cost-plus, called DRGs.

DRG, which stands for diagnosis related group, took various health problems (diagnoses) and lumped them together into groups for study of treatments and associated costs. For example, certain types of cancer may have been lumped into a group to study the treatments for these cancers and the costs associated with providing these treatments. Based on this review, a consistent, fixed payment price was established to reimburse providers of cancer care across the country, adjusted for urban and rural settings. Once the cost was determined, the government would pay that price to anyone treating a Medicare patient for this type of cancer—no more, no less.

In our broken finger example, Medicare would pay only 150 dollars. If the hospital's cost of fixing the finger was 100 dollars, it would make 50 dollars profit on the procedure. If the hospital's cost was 200 dollars, it would lose 50 dollars treating your finger.

For the first time, hospitals had to think about controlling costs. A hospital could end up losing money if it didn't get its costs in line. This sent shock waves through the industry. Providers complained bitterly about the cost pressures associated with the DRG system, while older Americans worried the quality of their care would suffer as hospitals began to slash costs.

But the system worked to reduce costs. Over the next ten years, the government became more and more strict about how they enforced DRGs. The number of treatments covered by DRGs increased, and the amount Medicare paid for these procedures decreased. For the first time in U.S. history, the percentage of increase in government health-care costs began to steady.

In the process, many providers began to feel the squeeze, especially those that primarily treated Medicare patients. Some hospitals even had to close their doors because they could not adapt to an environment that required a focus on cost control. Most providers, however, did adapt. They adapted through something called "cost shifting." Because they often lost money on Medicare patients, they shifted the cost of treating those patients to non-Medicare patients, charging them more than their treatment warranted.

Still, most Americans didn't care. Taxes were cut and employers still paid our health-care insurance premiums, which continued to rise to cover the cost shifting game. As consumers, we still had everything we wanted. We had the ability to choose any doctor or hospital, and the insurance company paid the bills in full.

But somewhere around 1992, things began to change. The government was now spending 14 percent of its budget dollars on health care, which translated into roughly 808 billion dollars. Political and financial pressures were at an all-time high to get this issue under control as projections called for government spending of 1.74 trillion dollars by the year 2000. The costs had exceeded all reasonable limits, and balancing the budget was quickly becoming an impossible task.

Additionally, as "downsizing" became a new word in corporate America, a number of people were forced out of work and lost their health insurance in the process. Although many people found new jobs, some companies no longer offered health-care benefits to new employees, or imposed pre-existing condition clauses and lengthy waiting periods until health benefits would be made available. Many people found themselves without health coverage for the first time.

Suddenly, the cost of health care made a difference. People without insurance began to realize just how expensive health care had become, and employers struggled with the skyrocketing cost of premiums. Those without insurance began to lobby Congress, making health care even more of a political issue. Large corporations began to negotiate for better rates with insurance companies and directly with local providers. As time passed, the health-care industry entered a mild state of chaos. No one completely understood what to do, but everyone knew somebody had to do something.

With all this activity, a young governor from Arkansas took center stage with his political platform for health-care reform. His ideas to reduce cost and gain universal access to health care for all Americans seemed to strike a chord with many voters. So in 1993, roughly ten years after DRGs were first introduced, health care once again became front page news.

The Clinton Years—And I Don't Mean Bill

Once President Bill Clinton named Hillary Clinton to head up a task force on health-care reform, the battle lines were drawn. Even the word "reform" implied the system was corrupt, or at least completely broken—putting the entire industry on the

defensive. The administration seemed intent on curbing the profits that doctors, hospitals and drug companies were making from
"helpless" Americans, while the providers and drug manufactur-
ers complained they were innocent victims in a ruthless political
attack. As usual, the motive was money. However, most of the
arguments had some truth to them, making the debate that followed much more confusing. No one group seemed to be
completely to blame for the problems, nor were they completely
blameless. Nor did they have one best solution to create a better
system. Consider the following positions each side took during
the deliberations:

- Health-care providers claimed they had been drained by
  DRGs and now were under attack by tough-minded employers.

- With so many people out of work, providers complained
  they were having to cover the cost of care for people who
  could not pay. In some cases (AIDS patients, for example),
  the bad debt could approach hundreds of thousands of dollars per patient.

- Providers also argued they had to pay huge premiums for
  liability insurance due to a legal system that awarded millions per case in malpractice.

- Pharmaceutical companies wanted people to understand the
  millions of dollars spent on research and development for
  new drugs. They threatened to stop that research if drug
  prices were going to be regulated by the government in any
  way. This, they argued, would slow down drug-related cures
  and force more expensive surgical intervention.

- Corporations claimed they could no longer bear the burden
  of health-care premiums that they were paying to cover the
  "losses" of DRG regulations. Smaller companies went out of
  business as a result of these cost increases, creating more
  unemployed, uninsured people.

- Both national and state governments argued they couldn't even consider balancing a budget with health-care costs as high as they were.

- Many Americans *without* insurance claimed they had lost their life savings because of illness. They demanded coverage for all Americans without pre-existing condition clauses, which came to be known as "universal access."

- Americans *with* insurance didn't want to lose what they had. They wanted full coverage and the option of going to whatever doctor or hospital they chose. A program with universal access might limit flexibility and decrease the quality of care received. The only way to provide care to everyone was to reduce care for some to increase care for others.

With all these divergent wants and needs, it's no wonder the Clintons didn't achieve what they set out to accomplish. But in my opinion, they accomplished a great deal. (And I'm a Republican!) They got America talking. And in the process, a new type of health care was born—managed care.

Managed Care

The word "manage" is defined as "to direct or control the use of." Up until this point, however, health care had neither controls nor direction. As we've seen, care was provided without thought to cost or (in some cases) need. If society was to begin to manage this care, some fundamental changes would need to be made in the system. Managed care would mean when care was provided:

- Costs should be an important consideration to all parties, not just to payors.

- Financial risk should be spread among consumer, provider and payor to encourage cost-conscious behavior of all parties.

- Treatment options should be considered by the consumer, provider and payor to discourage providers from treating more than necessary.

- More should not always mean better if a simple treatment would be as effective as a complex, high-tech treatment.

- Difficult decisions would have to be made based on whether the benefit to the patient and/or society no longer outweighs the cost of the care.

Managed care, or some other way to transform the system, became a subject of intense debate. Despite the controversy, some changes began to appear gradually throughout the country. Today more than half of the people who have insurance are covered under some type of managed care plan. Which type, however, depends on where you live. Some markets have been very aggressive in their attempts to curb costs, while others have moved much more slowly.

The most extreme form of managed care to date took shape along the lines of the DRG system, only on a much grander scale. Rather than regulate how much would be paid per procedure (as happened with DRGs), these managed care agreements decide how much will be paid per patient, no matter how many procedures are performed. This is known as a "managed life", or "capitation" (putting a "cap" on costs).

In these arrangements, the payors of health care pay the providers a fixed amount per person covered in their insurance plan. If a person never gets sick, the provider keeps all the money. If a person gets sick a lot, the provider has to bear the incremental financial burden. Thus providers make a lot of money if people stay well and lose a lot of money if they get sick.

The capitation system does many things:

1. It encourages providers to focus on wellness. Providers make money only if you stay *out* of the hospital, not *in* the hospital as with the cost-plus system. You may therefore notice

more programs focused on how to eat right, quit smoking, detect breast cancers earlier and so on.

2. It gets providers focused on cost. If you do end up in the hospital, the provider wants you out as soon as possible, with as few tests as possible to keep costs down. Remember, the provider now bears the burden of cost, not the payor.

3. It creates competition. As insurance companies take their huge volume of covered lives out to providers, the providers have to bid for that business. For example, if there are two hospitals in a market and an insurance company covers most of the people in that market, one hospital could win big with a contract and the other could lose big. In this case, each hospital will bid very aggressively to "win" those patients, or face possible extinction.

4. It creates restrictions. If an insurance company has negotiated a managed care contract with Hospital A, *you have to go to Hospital A*. If you go to Hospital B, you will not be covered and will be responsible for all charges.

Notice how the system aligns providers, payors and consumers. Providers can be very profitable if they control costs and keep their patients healthy. Payors make higher profits because they have shifted the financial risk to providers. And consumers can still get great coverage if they stay with the insurance company's network of providers. It's a system that can work for everyone.

Not all markets across the country, however, have gone this far. Some states and cities are still stuck in the cost-plus stage, while others have only begun to dabble in managed care. At the moment, most managed care arrangements center on a discount structure or fixed-fee arrangement. In these agreements, providers offer large discounts on the cost of care or a competitive flat rate per procedure, in return for the volume of patients each employer or insurance company can deliver. This leads to the same four "behavioral" changes listed above, except the financial risk to the provider is not as great, and therefore the insurance company needs to be more active in approving each procedure.

Regardless of where you live, managed care will likely become prevalent there. In the process, the flexibility you have as consumers to choose where you go for care will decrease. Doctors and hospitals will make less money, and the power base in health care will shift from the providers to the payors.

In the process, costs will go down. They already have. One study conducted by KPMG Peat Marwick, as reported in the February 12, 1996, issue of *Modern Healthcare*, showed hospital costs in managed care markets fell 11 percent below the national average. This same study found mortality rates were 5.25 percent below the national average as well. It seems quality improves.

If managed care is here to stay, we need to learn how to work within the system to get the best coverage for our children. In order to do that, we need to educate ourselves on the managed care options available to us.

Managed Care Options

Managed care now takes several forms. A review of these options, and a few definitions follow:

Definitions

Deductible—The amount you must pay before the insurance company pays anything. Deductibles are used by payors to help avoid paying out on every policy. Most people require only basic care, with minimal expense. With a deductible in place, the consumer pays for basic care and uses the insurance policy to avoid the risk of significant medical expenses.

Co-payment— A portion of cost you share with the insurance company each time you need care, after you have met your deductible requirement. A co-payment can be either a flat rate or a percentage of cost. For example, your co-payment might be 10 dollars every time you go to the doctor, or 20 percent of the cost of the care you receive while at the doctor's office.

Out-of-pocket expenses —These are the expenses the consumer is expected to pay. Out-of-pocket expenses typically equal the deductible amount plus co-payments. Many policies have out-of-pocket maximums in the event you incur extreme medical costs. Once the out-of-pocket maximum has been met, the policy begins to pay 100 percent of the cost of care.

Managed Care Choices

Although several other forms of managed care are emerging, the following four models represent the majority of managed care programs offered today.

Preferred Provider Organization (PPO)—The most common form of managed care at the time of this writing. PPO networks are created when employers or insurance companies (the payors) use their volume to leverage providers for deep discounts or competitive flat rates. The payors then "encourage" their members/employees to go to these preferred providers. This encouragement usually presents itself in the form of much better coverage from PPO providers, with lesser deductibles and co-payments. Paperwork is also greatly reduced because the payor and provider are linked together.

If a patient steps outside of this network, the penalties can be severe. The patient will pay a higher deductible, a higher co-payment and will be responsible for any amount over the discounted rate for medical treatment, which can be significant. The patient may also have to pay for the procedure up front and submit a claim for each invoice.

Health Maintenance Organization (HMO)—The first form of managed care (showing up as early as the 1960s), and they are the second most popular form of managed care in today's market. For the most part, HMOs cover both the financing and delivery of care because they are the payor and the provider. They tend to be the most cost-effective option but also the most strict. They typically allow little or no coverage outside of their network.

Point of Service (POS)—The fastest growing form of managed care today. The POS plan requires you to choose a primary care physician (PCP). The PCP has an arrangement with the insurance company to regulate the health-care choices you make and to ensure you use the preferred providers in their system. As a patient in this system, you must call or visit your PCP before making any health-care choices. The PCP will either attempt to treat you or will refer you to a specialist or hospital, each of which also has an arrangement with the insurance company. You must follow the directions of the PCP in order to receive coverage.

Exclusive Provider Organization (EPO)—A hybrid between an HMO and PPO that offers little or no coverage outside the preferred provider network.

Some Lingering Options

Despite the push toward managed care, other forms of health insurance are still available. These include:

Indemnity—This was the traditional form of coverage in years past and offered the most flexibility. A few companies still offer this option, but it is quickly becoming obsolete. As with most plans, coverage usually includes some form of deductible, co-payment and out-of-pocket maximum. You can go to any provider you choose, but you run the risk of going to a provider that charges more than what the payor considers "reasonable and customary." If your provider charges more than the payor's reasonable and customary limit, the payor will deduct that amount from the bill, leaving you responsible for the difference. (These limits were the insurance industry's first attempt to control costs.)

Say you had your gall bladder removed at a provider that charges 12,000 dollars for this procedure. You've already met your deductible, and your co-payment is set at 20 percent of cost. You expect to pay 2,400 dollars (20 percent of 12,000 dollars), but you find when you get your statement that you owe 4,000 dollars. What happened?

Your statement tells you the insurance company deducted 2,000 dollars from the total because the company's guidelines say 10,000 dollars are considered reasonable and customary for a gall bladder removal. Your insurance company then used the lesser figure to calculate its responsibility and paid the hospital 8,000 dollars (80 percent of 10,000 dollars). You then owe 4,000 dollars which includes the 2,000 dollars deducted for reasonable and customary limits and 2,000 dollar co-payment (20 percent of 10,000 dollars)

During Amanda's first year of treatment, these reasonable and customary charges cost our family more than 10,000 dollars in incremental payments, above and beyond deductibles and co-payments. The charges incurred over the reasonable and customary limits do not apply to the out-of-pocket maximums, so even though our maximum expense was supposed to be 5,000 dollars, it was really 15,000 dollars.

Self-Insured—Some large companies cover the risk of the cost of care themselves. Rather than pay out huge amounts to insurance companies, they put their own money aside to cover their employees if they become ill. The company is betting the care of those who become ill will cost less than the high premiums for each and every employee.

Catastrophic—Under these plans, some individuals gamble they won't get sick. They trade lesser premiums for a very high deductible—perhaps as high as 5,000 or 10,000 dollars. The consumers hope the cost of care they may require will be less than the premiums they would have had to pay out to receive better coverage.

Public Assistance Programs—These are programs such as Medicare and Medicaid. The Veteran's Affairs system of hospitals also provides free medical care to all veterans. There is no expense at all for any veteran who needs any kind of care.

Choosing the Best Health-Care Coverage

Finding and managing the best health coverage requires your direct involvement and active participation. Here are some pointers in finding and managing the best coverage:

- Be sure to examine all your options when looking for insurance. Although an HMO plan may be strict, if it covers the hospitals and doctors you need, it may be better than a more flexible PPO plan that does not cover the same providers.

- Interview your insurance companies. Talk to them about your child's condition. Do they have any restrictions such as pre-existing condition clauses that will prevent your child from getting the care he or she needs?

- Ask your doctors which insurance company they think provides the best coverage or plan. Find the plan that has the hospital you need in its network.

- If you don't have the flexibility to pick a plan that covers your hospital (most people don't), then work with your insurance company to see if an exception can be made. If your child needs specific care that cannot be provided at an in-network hospital, the insurance company may allow you to use your current hospital at full coverage.

- Ask your insurance company to assign you to a case manager. This is typically a nurse who is responsible for the most serious cases. By having one person who gets to know you and your child, it is easier to get your child admitted to the hospital or approved to see a specialist. Without one, every time your child needs care, you have to explain your child's case to someone who may not have an appreciation for how much you've been through or the seriousness of your child's condition. This is incredibly frustrating and can delay care while this new person reviews the case and seeks approval from supervisors who also don't know you or your child.

- Do everything you can to work within the system. If your insurance company sees you are a consumer who tries to keep costs down, it will be more likely to work with you on those rare occasions when you have to step outside the system. For example, when we went out of network for Amanda's liver transplant, we ran all her tests at an in-network hospital. Although this made our lives much more complicated, it also demonstrated our commitment to keep costs down.

- If you don't have insurance, work with the hospital's social workers. They can help you find the options for public assistance. They may be able to help you work out a payment plan.

- Whatever coverage you do (or don't) receive, make sure you understand your obligations. Communicate with your provider. If you're past due on a bill, call the provider and talk about it. It might help you with a payment plan or even give you a discount. Ignoring the bill will only make your provider more difficult to work with in the long run.

- Keep good records. Keep track of all your bills. (I still have every invoice dating back to 1992.) Match your charge slip together with your invoice, together with your insurance company's explanation of benefits. Watch for errors. In our case, about one out of every ten bills had an error of some kind on it, often overcharges or duplicate billings. Had I not kept good records, I never would have noticed this.

- If you identify an error, it is your responsibility to work it out. *Do not expect the provider and the insurance company to work it out for you.* They process thousands of bills each day.

The computer just keeps spitting out late notices until it automatically sends your bills to a collection agency.

- When resolving billing problems, make note of each conversation you have with the insurance company and provider. Jot down the person's name, as well as the date and time you spoke to him or her. Follow up these calls with a letter, along with copies of all the back-up documentation you have on file. You may have to repeat this process as many as five times over the course of several months before you can get even one problem resolved. It's like a full-time job, but if you don't get the billing issues resolved, they'll pile up until it is impossible to get out from under them.

- Take charge and take responsibility. Keep control of your finances so you can concentrate on your child's well-being. This is one of the issues that can overwhelm you. Don't let it.

- Don't be afraid to challenge a bill or the amount of the charge if you think it's wrong or excessive. As with any business, providers often charge as much as they can get. In a few cases, you can negotiate a better deal.

Don't give up. You *can* make it through the financial quagmire. If you have insurance, you may find many managed care programs actually make it easier to survive the financial burdens. With these programs, co-payments, deductibles and out-of-pocket expenses are greatly reduced. Paperwork is also reduced because you don't file a claim each time your child receives care. During the last two years, Amanda's care requirements have increased but our out-of-pocket expenses have been cut in half. Likewise, whereas I used to spend about twenty hours per week processing paperwork, I now spend about two.

What's Next With Managed Care?

During the two weeks it took me to write this chapter, I saw eight newspaper articles on managed care, three TV news reports, two magazine articles and one debate on the Internet. Each of these fourteen reports helped to clarify one thing— everyone has a different but very passionate opinion on how health care should be delivered in this country.

Some think health care is a right, while others don't understand why they should have to pay more so people who are out of work can have coverage. Some think we should have a full range of coverage with a multitude of options, while others would be happy with more restrictive, universal coverage. Some think we should save lives at all costs, while others contend we should let the "hopeless" die quickly so we can spend the money on those who could live more productive lives.

It's easy for those who have never faced illness to cast judgment on those of us who have lived with it. Our experience, however, often makes us blind to good judgment because we are caught up in the emotions of saving the lives of our children. Obviously, neither side can rationally make the right call on what the system should and should not offer.

I speak only for myself. Heroic recovery at any cost, financial and otherwise, has never been my goal. I believe peace and joy are found in the quality of life not the length of life. I'm not as concerned about extending Amanda's life as I am with making it wonderful while she's here. When Amanda decides it's time to go, she's going to go. And neither I nor the doctors will be able to do anything about it. At that time, aggressive medical therapy may only extend the suffering and add stress to the final days of her life.

In the meantime, I can measure the success of Amanda's care against the cost of her care very easily; I measure it in terms of laughter. As I write this paragraph, Amanda is running around upstairs and laughing with her sister. It's wild laughter, the kind that can be found only in the joyful play of children. It rings throughout the house as a beacon of hope. Just try to manage that!

---

1. Susan Brink and Rit Rubin, *U.S. News and World Report*, July 24, 1995, p. 60.

CHAPTER 5

Learning From Our Children

"Truly I tell you, whoever does not receive the kingdom of God as a little child will never enter in it."

—Luke 18:17

Journal Entry: June 1994

As I watch Amanda fight for her life, I think back to the event that brought us to the hospital just two short months ago.

It was an unusually warm day for an April in Chicago, so we got the bicycles out to take Missy (our dog) for a run around the neighborhood. I expected to put Amanda in the kids' seat on the back of my bicycle, but to my surprise she asked to try her own bike instead. Though it still had training wheels on it, this was a big step for her. She had spent the last three summers in the hospital and never had much time to ride it, nor did she ever seem to have the energy to go very far on her own.

So I got her helmet on and off we went. Sarah, as usual, took off at record speed. She was all the way down the street before Amanda and I even left the driveway. Amanda went very slowly but surely off on her maiden journey around the block. I tried to stay somewhere between the two girls in case

61

any cars came along. I could see Sarah up ahead and kept looking back to see if Amanda was okay. Each time she would wave and say she was fine. She looked so determined to make it on her own, and every time I offered to help, she refused. I was very proud of her for trying so hard and was equally as delighted that she was struggling to learn something all "normal" children have to learn on their own.

When we were almost completely around the block, I sent Sarah and Missy on to the house and returned to see how our little one was doing. As I came over the slight hill, I saw that she had gotten off the bicycle for the first time and was walking it home next to her. And when she saw me, she stopped. As I approached I could see that she was holding back tears. I assumed she was upset that she hadn't made it all the way home on the bicycle, but then I realized that there was something much more to this moment. She looked at me intently for about thirty seconds, trying to decide what she was going to say; I gave her the time to figure it out. Finally, with a cracked voice, she said, "Daddy, my 'beeper' (heart) hurts. It's been hurting me for a long time."

Instantly, I was sick to my stomach. I knew that this was not an excuse for not making it all the way on the bicycle. Instead, this was Amanda finally deciding it was time to tell me that something was not right inside of her. The few tears that she let go were not tears of wounded pride, but more the recognition that she could not deny the pain any longer. Something was wrong and she needed help.

I got off my bicycle and went to her side. I placed my hand on her chest and could feel her heart beat. It was extremely fast and very irregular. It felt as though she had about six different hearts beating inside her at the same time. I offered to carry her home, but she refused. She got back on the bike and rode the rest of the way by herself. When we got home, she went to bed and slept for about twenty hours straight.

Sarah went off to play with other friends. Deborah and I prepared to enter the maze one more time.

Of all my memories, this is one of the most vivid. I don't think I will ever forget the look on her face as she struggled to speak those words. How long she must have thought about letting us know that she was in pain, that it was time to go back to the doctor, that we hadn't yet completed this journey, that she needed us to carry her along just a little while longer. She apparently needed time to deal with it herself before letting us know. How complex this life for such a little girl.

Journal Entry: May 1995

"Do it again, Daddy. Do it again!"

I had played this game at least one hundred times in the last thirty minutes—the old make-the-penny-disappear-and-find-it-in-her-ear trick. The problem is that I'm not that good at it, and she already knows how it works. Making it seem like real magic gets harder with each turn. She watches my hand closely and doesn't let me distract her anymore.

As usual, we were in a hospital, waiting in some hallway for yet another ultrasound. It had been forty-five minutes since they sent us to radiology and we were getting anxious about what they would find. But then again, we knew what they would find. The CT Scan had already shown the cancer was back; in fact it had spread all over her body. Now we were just waiting to see how badly it had damaged her heart. I looked over to Deborah and she had that empty look. No emotion. No sadness. No tears. Just empty.

"Do it again, Daddy. Do it again!"

"Okay, Okay. But this is the last time."

I didn't have the energy for this. In fact, I didn't understand why Amanda was being so playful. I knew that she heard the conversation with the doctor on the way over here. I knew that she knew what was going on. Why wasn't she asking her usual batch of questions about what they were going to do to her? At the very least, why wasn't she complaining vigorously about having to go through yet another test? Instead, she seemed happier than she'd been in a long while. It stood in such contrast to the way I was feeling. It was making it difficult for me to concentrate.

"Do it again, Daddy. Do it again."

So I told her to say the magic words and blow on the coin for good luck. I tickled her cheek to create the distraction, but she knew better. She saw the coin fall into my other hand and took great pleasure in letting me know that she had caught me.

"I see it! I see it! It's in your other hand!"

I attempted to play "pretend" upset that she had caught me, but the real upset came through instead. "I have no magic left, Amanda," I said, though I wasn't talking about the penny. I put my head to the side to keep her from seeing my expression, but she took her hand to my cheek and pulled my face back around. She looked me right in the eye and said, "That's okay, Daddy. I still believe in magic, even if I can see the coin fall." She wasn't talking about the penny either. This child knows more than I think.

Journal Entry: August 1995

Deborah and the girls were driving back home from a trip to Florida when they passed by a graveyard. Very calmly, Amanda asked Deborah if there was a grave back in Chicago with her name on it. "No," said Deborah, "I don't think there is." But Amanda replied back as calmly as the first time, "Yes, Mommy, there's a grave back in Chicago with my name on it."

Learning From Our Children

This morning kicked off one week alone with the girls as Deborah headed to Florida for a college reunion. My first job as Mr. Mom was to give Amanda her oral chemotherapy before breakfast because she's supposed to take it on an empty stomach. I was a little frazzled trying to balance giving her medicine along with the preparation of French toast while simultaneously having a conversation with my girls. (This is a father's equivalent to chewing bubble gum and walking at the same time.) Nevertheless, I reached into the cabinet and grabbed two of her many medications, took out the required nine pills (six of one, three of another) and handed them to her.

She stared down at the tablets, rolled her eyes and looked at me with a smirk. Soon I realized I hadn't given her any milk, so I quickly poured a cup and handed it to her. She grabbed six of the pills, put them all in her mouth, took a sip of milk and down they went. (Amanda has been able to swallow very large numbers of pills since she was three.) But she did not take the other three pills. Once again she sat there, this time with a pretend disgusted expression, rolling her eyes and whispering to her sister. Finally I asked what was going on, and she said, "Daddy, these three are anti-nausea pills. I only take these if I feel sick to my stomach. The chemo pills I need are white, big and round. They're in a yellow bottle over there. Geeeeeez." Then both she and Sarah broke out in laughter that seemed to last a good ten minutes.

I smiled, both out of embarrassment and a realization of how knowledgeable this six-year-old girl is about such a complex set of circumstances. She continually surprises me about how aware she is of her situation. At age three she could tell us the proper sequence of IV chemotherapy drugs with saline and heparin. At age four she could detail what the emergency room staff would want to do at each visit. In fact, she'd often get annoyed at the doctors as they'd try to explain what they wanted to do. "I know, I know," she'd say. "Just do it and get it over with." By the time she was five, her vocabulary included the proper usage of terms such as CAT scan, liver transplant, surgery, spinal tap, chemo, ultrasound and hep-lock, which is what they do to your IV to keep the line from clotting when they remove you from the intravenous fluids. Now, at six, she is able to tell us if she needs pain medication to get through a rough night. She can tell us if she needs to go see a doctor or if she just needs to get some rest. She's an active participant in her own care and regularly helps us to help her.

But Amanda is more than just a little technologically advanced. She is also very intuitive relative to how *we* feel about her illness. She seems to be able to pick out our saddest moments and offer a perspective that helps us better understand how to find some meaning in it all. Sometimes she's able to offer us humor to diffuse a tense moment. Other times she offers a peek into the mind of God to help us see why we might be going through all of this misery. Most of the time, however, she's experiencing sadness or joy, just like Deborah and me— feeling these feelings right alongside of us; not apart from us.

I remember one afternoon I got a call at work from Deborah who had rushed Amanda to the ER earlier that morning. The doctors were going to have to admit Amanda and I needed to stay with her at the hospital because Deborah had not been able to pack any clothes before she left. I went home, packed and started the two-hour trek downtown. When I arrived, they were still in the ER because no rooms were available (you can wait all day for a bed to open up at the bigger medical centers). Amanda had been stabilized and was sitting on a stretcher, hooked up to an IV, an EKG and pulse-oximeter. She looked so fragile.

Deborah and I caught up on the latest news from the doctor, and then she gathered her coat to leave. Amanda sat up to say good-bye and watched her mommy walk out of the ER. I closed the exam room door and suddenly found myself feeling incredibly depressed. We had been in the hospital an average of two weeks out of every four for the last five months, and I was tired of having our family constantly ripped apart. Now once again we'd be separated for another two weeks. I felt the tears starting to come, but tried to push them back. I looked over at Amanda and saw she also was trying to hold them back.

My instinct was to be strong for her since the last thing Amanda needed was for me to fall apart. She had a rough two weeks ahead and needed to know that I'd be there for her. But then she looked at me and asked, "Are you going to cry, Daddy?" I replied, "I think so." "Me too," she whispered back. Then we both let the tears go. We held each other and cried; not for long but enough so we let our real feelings flow. Soon we both were fine. We sat silently for another fifteen minutes or so, and then started to play our familiar hospital games. We even had moments when we could laugh every now and then. She had been my release and I was hers. That moment gave us both the strength we needed to get through the rigors of the next two weeks.

I find both strength and peace in Amanda all the time. I learn from her every day. Although she may not realize it, she helps support the family as much as we support her. But it wasn't always so mutually beneficial; we have achieved this relationship slowly over the past four years. In the early stages of her illness, we couldn't look to her for help and support. She's just a child, after all, and a sick one at that, we told ourselves. She needs to be protected and shielded from the trauma of her illness. Amanda needs us to be strong. Don't let her see you cry or be sad. Don't tell her about what she's about to face. And whatever you do, don't let her know she might die.

But ultimately, shielding your child from his or her illness is unfair to everyone. For one thing, it prevents your child from participating in the most important thing affecting his or her life; and it denies you the opportunity of finding strength and knowledge from your child's insight. A mother of a child with AIDS once said she thought God planted a lifetime of wisdom in her little five-year-old. I think that's true of many kids who are seriously ill. How sad it would be if we were to lose the benefit of that wisdom because we thought we knew better than they did, or that only we could bear the weight of the burden.

By allowing ourselves to rely on our children, we can learn from them. At the same time, we can help them to deal with their illness. In order to establish this kind of relationship, however, we must make a conscious effort to do two things: talk to our kids and listen to them.

Sounds pretty simple doesn't it? But there's nothing simple about it. At least not at first. Learning how to talk to your children about his or her possible death, or explaining why he or she is different from other kids can seem like an impossible task. Likewise, listening to them and involving them goes against every parental instinct to protect, nurture and teach. Nevertheless, for those who persevere, a mutually beneficial relationship can be found. Let's take a look.

To Tell the Truth—Talking to Our Kids

Throughout the early stages of treatment, you will establish an important communication link with your child. As the whirlwind of activity begins to swirl around you, you will hear the quiet (and sometimes not so quiet), questioning voice of your child asking you to explain why all this is happening. As you attempt to answer this question, you will establish in your child's mind and your own, a level of trust that will become the foundation for your communication throughout the illness.

Consider the following example: A father takes his son to the hospital for a spinal tap. The boy asks if the needle will hurt and because the father doesn't want his son to worry he says, "No." But of course the needle *does* hurt. One week later, the boy needs to go to the hospital for a follow-up exam. There will be no needles this time, so the father tells the boy it won't hurt.

The boy wants to believe his dad, but all he remembers is that the needle in his back hurt when his father said it wouldn't and all day he worries about the exam, his stress level building. As the day progresses, the father can't understand why the boy is acting out. They fight off and on during the entire visit to the hospital, and the son says he wants his mother to take him to the doctor the next time. The father is deeply hurt. From that point on, he isn't sure how to help his son through the struggle. They eventually stop communicating with each other because it is too painful to talk about the illness without a level of trust.

What should this father have done? Not tell his son about the hospital visit at all? No, because if there is a sudden surprise visit to the doctor, he'll ultimately begin to wonder if he's ever safe. He'll never know if he can relax, or if Mom and Dad are going to "take me in." The best course would be for the father to tell his son he has to go to the hospital for a spinal tap and leave it at that. If, however, his son asked a question about the needle, the father should answer honestly, "Yes, the needle will hurt. But it will only last a few seconds and I'll be there with you the entire time."

The boy may worry about the procedure initially, but at least he knows exactly what lies ahead and can spend some time mentally preparing, just as adults appreciate the chance to prepare for major events in their lives. Although these first few trips to the hospital may be traumatic for the whole family, the trust you establish far outweighs the benefits of a few hours of peace you may gain by keeping your child in the dark.

During the first year of Amanda's illness, we struggled with how to communicate with her. We wouldn't discuss anything around her, and when she had to go to the hospital we waited until the last minute to tell her. We thought we were protecting her from all the pressures, but we actually created more stress. She expected the worst and soon began to think of us as part of the problem. She panicked during every procedure, no matter how many times we told her there were no "owies" involved. She eventually stopped talking to us altogether.

Eventually, however, we began to include her in our discussions about her treatment. If something was going to hurt, we told her so—if she asked. If she had to go in for surgery or another major procedure, we told her several days in advance. This gave her a couple of days to think of questions and to prepare for it. Although she did worry about it a little (as any of us would), she began to trust we had told her everything and there would be no additional surprises. She knew exactly what to expect and could determine what fell within her ability to deal with the pain and aggravation. As a result, she could put it out of her mind, play with her friends and have fun right up until the day she had to go to the hospital.

Even on days she was scheduled to be admitted to the hospital, she managed to maintain a positive outlook. On the morning of her second heart surgery to remove some tumor mass, she came downstairs with a big smile and said, "Today is bald day!" (realizing chemotherapy would also begin that night). I was a wreck, but she was as upbeat as any other day of the week. She told me although she wasn't allowed to eat anything, it was OK if I had breakfast since I might get hungry while she was in surgery. I can't imagine what would have happened if we had waited until that morning to tell her what was going to happen.

We had told her about the surgery a week earlier. When we explained to her that she needed to go back to the hospital for an operation and chemo, she started to cry and became very depressed. Within a day, she became quiet and withdrawn. We were unsure how much more to share with her, but then we finally decided to tell her why it was so important for her to go back to the hospital. For the first time ever, we told her if we didn't do this, she might die.

We had denied death for a long time. Two years earlier when a child at school had told her she was going to die, we told her absolutely not, and the topic never came up again. The subject of death seemed to be too much for any child to bear, and so it was for Amanda. But her condition was so serious this time, we felt we had to tell her. And when we did, it seemed as though she already knew; now it was just confirmed.

I'll never forget her expression when we told her. Her eyes went from empty to intensely contemplative. She stared at us for a few seconds and then looked at her stomach and chest. We had explained where all the tumors were and she seemed to be thinking about what they must look like inside of her. Then her whole face lit up. She looked back at us and said, "OK, whatever you think is best." She got up and went over to the mirror and pulled her hair back to picture herself bald again. "I hate being bald," she said. "Can I call Laura and go outside to play?"

And that was it. Painful as it was, honest communication helped Amanda understand why we had to move forward. Anything less would have led to a breakdown in our relationship—or at least a huge wedge between us. As things turned out, we needed our closeness more than ever because the next two months would be the most difficult time so far. We needed every ounce of love and trust to make it through that time and come out intact as a family.

In many ways, I'm grateful we had time to learn how to handle these tough situations before we encountered more difficult ones. Had the need for a third round of chemotherapy come up earlier, we wouldn't have known how to gauge Amanda's readiness to hear the devastating news, nor would we have been able to draw upon her strength at a time when we really needed it.

Listening to Our Children

As you may have sensed by now, our ability to communicate with Amanda evolved over time. At first we were deceptive with her about her situation; then we told her just enough to be truthful. Eventually we included her in all aspects of her care. One of the reasons we were able to establish a more open relationship was we matured as parents. Another reason was we sensed Amanda was prepared to hear the information. She had learned from her experiences it was better to know what was going to happen to her rather than be surprised. She also grew more comfortable with her condition and the medical environment in which she often lived, which helped her absorb more of the information. As with most things, she was able to handle more over time.

I am not recommending "full disclosure" at first, especially if your child is very young. Even to this day, we break the news to Amanda gradually about certain issues. Sometimes saying just enough to be truthful is the right thing to do. The trick is to pick up on the clues your child sends you to determine what he or she is ready to hear or would rather avoid. Deborah and I have discovered by listening closely to Amanda, we can piece together the clues to determine her readiness for just about anything.

The key is listening. It will help you determine how to care for your child, and will help you pick up on his or her emotional *and* physical needs. Listening, however, involves more than just hearing the words your child says to you. It means watching how he or she behaves and talks to siblings or friends. Above all, it means hearing what your child *doesn't* say.

For example, your child may not know how to express something, or may not understand enough about what's happening to even know something's wrong. If a child has never had a healthy body, he or she may assume that pain or discomfort is a natural state. Your child may not tell you something doesn't feel right because he or she has always felt that way. You have to be "listening" to determine what's really going on.

When we first learned Amanda was in need of a liver transplant, we couldn't believe it. She hadn't been on chemo for almost six months and she seemed so normal. We told the doctor he must be wrong because she looked too good to be near liver failure. But then he began to talk about how she was compensating for her illness, and we just didn't see it. He said she probably preferred coloring pictures to playing sports. That she probably liked being alone more than being with other kids. And that she probably slept more than our other daughter. He was right. She had been compensating for her poor health. It wasn't that she didn't like other kids, she just couldn't keep up.

The same goes for her emotional behavior. Amanda's bad moods are not always due to the drugs she takes or to normal kid stuff. Often she is masking how upset she is at her condition. When she told us recently she doesn't like school, she was really upset over something far more serious. Over the course of a twenty-minute conversation, we learned the older kids tease her about being bald. This led to a question as to why the chemo makes her hair fall out, which led to the real reason she was feeling upset—she has cancer and other kids don't. Had we dismissed her feelings and said, "Of course you like school," we never would have gotten to the heart of what she really wanted to say.

But these conversations are not just for her benefit; I learn from them as well. During this same discussion, I learned Amanda doesn't care about the kids teasing her because she knows her hair will grow back and thinks anyone who teases her isn't worth worrying about. (Isn't that a lesson from which we can all benefit?!) I also found out that while she is very sad about her cancer, she believes when she goes to heaven, she won't have any of these problems any more, so why worry about it now? Upon hearing this, I began to wonder if she was talking about her feelings, or if God was sending a message to me about how I should be feeling. Either way, I walked away a better man. This kind of thing happens *all the time.*

Despite all the wisdom, Amanda is a child after all. Like all children, she waffles back and forth from tenacious to timid, from strong to delicate and from fighter to fainthearted. As her parents, we've discovered a kind of code that lets us know what she wants. When she asks questions about what's going on with her treatment, she wants honest answers and a chance to participate in the decision-making process. When she doesn't ask about it, she doesn't want to deal with her illness at that moment; instead she wants us to bear the weight of the burden and tell her what to do. She's also looking for us to be strong at that time, not to share our sorrows, confusion or discomfort, but to lead her through the pain with grace and strength—sometimes for a very long time, even months.

As with everything, we look for the balance. We are open with Amanda, but only to the extent she is prepared for the facts. We share our sadness, but only to the extent she wants to know our real feelings. We are honest with bad news, but only to the extent she has had enough time to absorb the little things first. We talk to her, but only to the extent we have listened first and know what she needs and wants to hear.

You can have a wonderful, trusting relationship with your child, even as you go through the trauma of illness. Listen for clues from your child as to what he or she needs from you. Be strong when they need it, but let your child be strong for you as well. Those few times you let your guard down may be the times you grow the closest together and share the deepest peace. You *can* find strength in the heart of a little child.

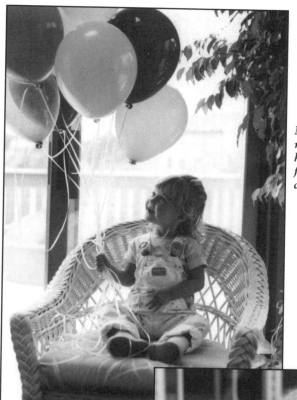

May 1991: Amanda returns home from the hospital after her very first surgery and first chemo treatment.

June 1991: Amanda during her first round of chemo.

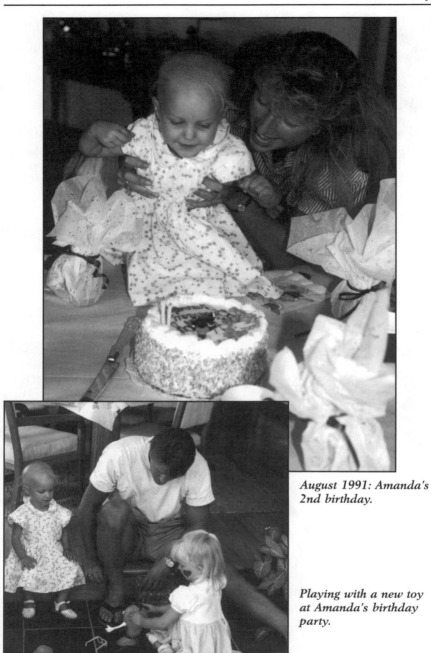

*August 1991: Amanda's
2nd birthday.*

*Playing with a new toy
at Amanda's birthday
party.*

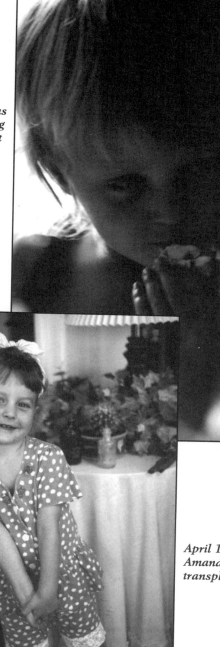

August 1992: 3rd birthday. Amanda's hair has grown back during the end of her first round of chemo. You can see her tired eyes.

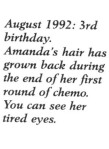

April 1993: Before Amanda's liver transplant.

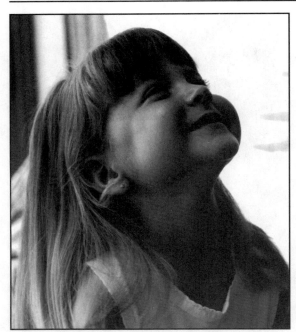

May 1994: The day Amanda was diagnosed with Lymphoma—the first time.

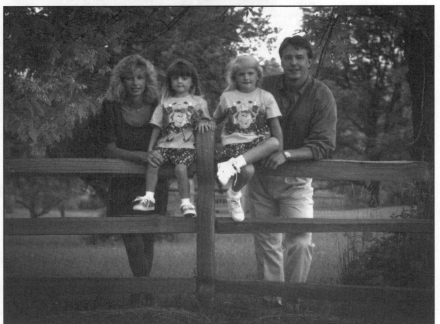

May 1994: One week after Amanda was diagnosed with Lymphoma. We thought this would be our last family picture. Amanda has a fever of 105° at the time this picture was taken.

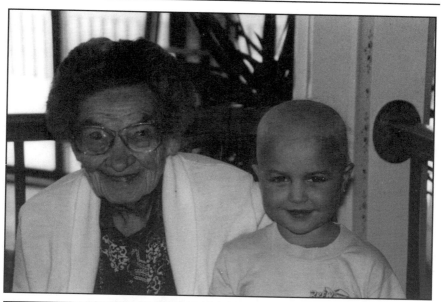

Amanda and her great-grandmother.

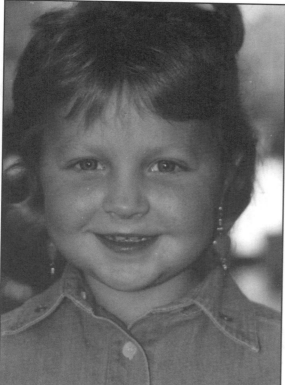

May 1995: Amanda's hair grows back after her second round of chemo. Her face is somewhat swollen from aggressive use of steriods.

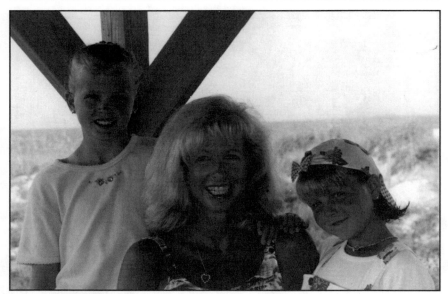

July 1997: Deborah and the girls.

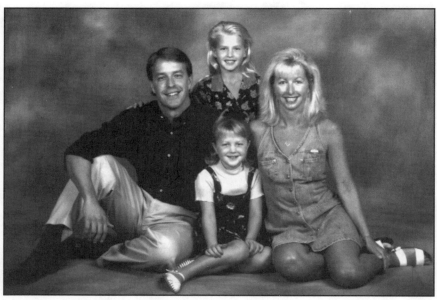

September 1997: Family portrait.

CHAPTER 6

What About Me?
—The Siblings

"What about me, what about me?!"

—Sarah MacLellan

A Letter to Sarah: June 1991

Dear Sarah,

I'm staying at the Ronald McDonald House tonight because the hospital will let only one parent sleep in the room with Amanda. The other parents staying here are very nice, but they speak so matter-of-factly about their children's illnesses. How can it be so casual for them? Don't they know this is devastating?!

I miss you, Sarah. You're my friend and I need friends right now. But you're far away. Grandpa and Mima say you're being very good. You went to their house in Flat Rock four days ago so we could care for Amanda during this very difficult time. Your Grandpa flew to Chicago to pick you up on Father's Day. He didn't know what to say, but he tried very hard to give me the love I needed. He did.

After our brief visit, they made the final call for the flight back to North Carolina. There wasn't a ramp leading out to the plane, so you had to walk outside and down some stairs. I stood at the window looking down at you. You turned around and looked up at me with your precious smile. I

81

waved and you waved back. My hand stayed up and touched upon the glass. Slowly my forehead touched the glass as well. I never needed you so much. It was Father's Day and my child was leaving, as was my own father. Three generations caught in a new struggle.

Just before you entered the plane, you turned and waved again. I didn't move. I couldn't. You're only three years old. You shouldn't be going through this either. I love you.

Journal Entry: January 1992

Sarah has become much more aware of Amanda's situation. She understands now that her sister's sickness is different from a cold or tummy ache. She's been to the hospital with us for Amanda's chemo treatments and I watch her watch the other kids. Some of them look so horrible. Sarah looks at them and then looks at Amanda. She's not sure what to think.

Journal Entry: July 1994

Today is the first holiday in more than a year that Amanda has not been in the hospital. I took the girls to a parade this morning and had a blast. As I watched them play, I realized that my greatest regret about this whole situation is that Sarah and Amanda have lost so much of their childhood together. This last hospitalization really highlighted the contrast in their lives: While Sarah went to a birthday party this past week, Amanda was in surgery; while Sarah played in the summer sun, Amanda was getting bone marrow samples taken out of her hip. Their lives are taking them in such very different directions, and I miss their closeness. I miss our closeness.

Journal Entry: November 1994

As I look back on this journal, I see that there is someone who gets much too little attention—my Sarah. She's a vic-

tim too, and she handles it better than all of us. She is such a good girl. She is loving when Amanda is sick. She is understanding when pulled from her bed in the middle of the night and shipped off to a neighbor's house. She is playful and childlike, even in such a grown up situation.

Sarah, I want you to know that you are an inspiration to me. I look to you for guidance when my spirit is weak. Your childlike trust and fascination remind me of what Christ asks us to be like in the Bible. I learn a lot from you and thank you for all that you are.

Journal Entry: April 1995

The simplicity of children is glorious. I watch outside my window where Sarah and Amanda are flying kites in the sunshine. Amanda sits quietly and lets the wind do the work, while Sarah finds joy in helping the kite by running wildly around the yard. This simple act speaks volumes about their personalities and styles. I find myself comparing them, but then ask myself, "Why compare?" They represent the full spectrum of childhood—wonder and amazement, energy and excitement. I am so grateful to be part of their lives. My cup runneth over.

Journal Entry: May 1995

I sat out on the deck tonight to watch the sun set. Sarah was playing with the neighborhood kids, and I watched her run free for awhile. Amanda lay sleeping just inside the house on the couch in the sun room; she was having a tough night.

I called Sarah home to watch the last of the brilliant colors fade to gray. I picked her up and placed her on my lap and embraced her. After a few minutes of silence, I told her that Amanda was sick again and that we had to take her back to the hospital for more surgery and chemotherapy.

She asked questions about what was wrong, how long would it be, was Amanda OK—and then, who would be taking care of her while we were gone? We talked about all the details of the next few days and then spent some time watching the night sky begin to take shape. I realized how much I missed these moments with her when we were apart and I told her so. I told her that one of the saddest things of all for me was that I couldn't spend as much time with her as I wanted to. I told her that I was sorry that she was always left behind and that we have to spend so much time taking care of Amanda.

Without hesitation, she looked at me and said, "That's OK, Daddy. Amanda's sick and she needs more of your attention. I'm OK, I have my friends. You need to take care of Amanda."

I had no response, only admiration.

We sat there until the last of the gray sky turned black and then headed inside. Amanda was moaning in her sleep. Sarah walked over to her and stared for a while. She found a blanket, covered her up and then began to rub her back.

This whole thing is just so unfair.

Journal Entry: August 1995

I went to check on the girls after they had gone to bed tonight. I stood there for several minutes watching them sleep. As usual, Amanda had gotten out of her bed to sleep with Sarah. While I watched, Amanda let out a groan, as she does all night long. And without hesitation, Sarah turned over, stretched out her hand and rubbed her head. Amanda leaned into Sarah and they partially embraced. All of this happened without either one waking up. How deep their love must be that they tend to each other's needs while sleeping.

What About Me?—The Siblings

This chapter tells the story of how my oldest daughter, Sarah, is affected by Amanda's illness. Although Sarah is one of the most precious gifts any parent could receive, she's getting only one chapter out of an entire book on Amanda. That's the way it seems to end up at home—Sarah gets about 10 percent of the attention. It's not a fifty-fifty deal; it never has been and probably never will be.

If there's anything I feel guilty about in my life, it's that a wonderful, beautiful, loving child like Sarah sometimes feels second in importance to Amanda's illness. Just as Amanda doesn't deserve her lot in life, neither does Sarah. While she handles it all very well, it's still hard for her to deal with all of this.

The challenges faced by the siblings of sick kids are burdensome but often not fully appreciated by their parents, who have temporarily shifted into a survival mode. The issues for these siblings range from simple, ego-based dilemmas, to more complex, stress-related anxiety. As I have thought about some of the factors that impact Sarah in our household, I have come to realize just how much she has been affected by Amanda's illness. For example:

- Sarah loves her sister very much. In fact, Amanda is her best friend. She worries about her well-being just as much as we do and is just as distressed about Amanda's condition as we are during some of the most difficult times.

- We constantly have to ship Sarah off to neighbors during emergencies, often in the middle of the night. Her life is in a constant state of flux, and she is never completely sure where she might end up when Amanda goes to the hospital.

- Although we always try to make sure at least one parent is with her at big events such as grade school graduations and recitals, we miss a lot of these occasions when Amanda is sick.

- Since Amanda is often too ill to eat or do chores or school-work, it seems to Sarah that we have a double standard with our expectations and house rules.

- When Amanda gets ill, she requires virtually 100 percent of our attention. Sarah is usually sent off to play somewhere else, often by herself.

- Although we try to make plans to do fun things with Sarah, we often have to cancel due to emergency medical issues. She may get excited about something for weeks, only to be disappointed at the very last minute.

- Amanda often gets presents and cards from kind people who want to do something nice for her while she's in the hospital. It's hard for Sarah to see her sister lavished with gifts while she doesn't get anything.

- Nothing Sarah does seems to compare to the drama of Amanda's life. When people meet our girls, they have a tendency to focus on Amanda. They also see her bald head or swollen face (from the steroids) and try extra hard to make her feel pretty. Although Deborah and I appreciate the extra effort and attention aimed at Amanda, it makes Sarah feel like she can't compete.

As Sarah's parents, Deborah and I also fall into some traps that make life more confusing and stressful for her. In the early stages of Amanda's illness, we stumbled into these pitfalls without even being aware of them. As time passed, we realized where the traps lay and tried to avoid them, but would get snared nonetheless. Over the years, however, we've learned how to elude most of them. While issues differ for every family, ours presented themselves as follows:

- By the time we finish tending to Amanda, Deborah and I are exhausted. It's hard to find the energy to be "up" for Sarah even though she deserves our enthusiastic attention.

- When we're tired, we are less able to tolerate the normal, everyday challenges of parenting; consequently we are sometimes much harder on Sarah than we would be without all the stress and sleep deprivation.

- After going through a day of painful procedures with Amanda, it's easy to forget how important it is to make a big deal over Sarah's scraped knee, bee sting or whatever. It seems to Sarah we don't care about her pain, only Amanda's.

- It's often hard to discipline Amanda because she's been through so much pain in her life. It's easy to let her get away with things we would discipline Sarah for, thus creating a double standard.

- Deborah and I have an overriding insecurity about losing Amanda. As a result, we try to fit a lifetime of love and living into each day with her. Sometimes we find ourselves waiting until Amanda is gone to focus on Sarah. But Sarah should not have to put her life on hold for five or ten years while Amanda gets all our love and attention. Otherwise, it will leave her asking, "What about me?!"

Bonding With the Siblings

Despite all of this, Sarah is incredibly well adjusted. God gave us all a gift when he gave her an independent spirit and a gregarious personality that allows her to make friends quickly. He also gave her a loving soul, which helps her to put Amanda first despite a natural childhood tendency to want everything just for herself. These traits have enabled her to adjust to our family situation more easily.

In fact, Sarah's strength has made it easier for all of us to adjust. I'll be forever grateful to her for being so mature at such a young age, but at the same time I'll always appreciate how much she has taught me about having a childlike spirit. She is so enthusiastic, so playful, so faithful about a positive outcome for everything it is impossible to walk away from her without some of that joy rubbing off. Her playful spirit is contagious.

Perhaps as a result of Sarah's faithful nature, Deborah and I have gotten better about balancing Amanda's illness with everything else in our lives. We've been able to let go of some of the pain and some of the constant worry in order to think about things other than sickness. One of the first things we were able to think about was how to better meet Sarah's needs. (Give some joy and get some back!) After all, she needs to feel special, loved and equally as important as any other member of the family.

As with any relationship, re-bonding with Sarah required hard work and concentration. The first step was to make sure we steered clear of the traps mentioned above; they were damaging Sarah's self esteem and required immediate correction. Once we reversed the negative ways in which we were dealing with her, we considered a few additional steps to boost her spirit and make her feel even more important to us and to the family as a whole:

- We make sure Sarah is an active part of Amanda's health care. We are as open and honest with her about Amanda's illness as we are with Amanda. We take Sarah to the hospital so she can see what happens there, and we ask Sarah to help with some of the home care, which sometimes means "just" holding Amanda's hand. This way, Sarah feels as though she is *part* of the process, not *outside* of it.

- Although we're honest with Sarah about what's happening, we also let her know she need not worry about Amanda. We've told her to care about her sister and to tend to her needs when she can, but she should leave the worry to Mommy, Daddy and especially God.

- We've told her it's OK to be happy and have fun when Amanda's sick. She should not feel guilty about being a normal kid.

- We've also told her it's OK to be sad about her sister, and she should share those feelings with us or with Amanda.

- We make sure both Sarah and Amanda realize every gift sent to Amanda really is for both of them, since they are both affected by everything associated with a hospital visit. Now they're both excited when the presents come.

- Sarah and Amanda receive equal reward and equal discipline, which is just as important for Amanda as it is for Sarah. Sarah now sees this and at least feels the rules are fair.

- Whenever possible, we try to give Sarah special attention. Sometimes this involves a special event; other times, it's nothing more than an extra long hug. While this never completely balances the time we spend with Amanda, Sarah knows she can count on our full attention at least part of the time.

- Most important, we make sure Sarah has every opportunity just to be a kid. Even though Amanda doesn't have a normal childhood, Sarah shouldn't be penalized for it. She is involved in Girl Scouts, gymnastics, ballet and other activities. She plays with friends, goes to birthday parties and participates in school activities, even during the most challenging times. Although it often hurts Amanda deeply to see her sister run off to do things she is not able to do herself, it would be unfair to hold Sarah back.

While all of this has gone a long way toward improving Sarah's perspective on Amanda's illness, we still have our fair share of issues with her. On occasion she cries, complains and is totally disruptive to the family to get attention. Sometimes she's distant and contemptuous of us when we return home from an extended hospital stay. At other times she's despondent and depressed when she misses out on some fun activity due to a medical emergency. And she will exploit anything that happens to her (a bump, a scrape, etc.) for weeks at a time, demanding as much indulgence as we provide Amanda during her tough times.

However, we found none of these issues to be so challenging they can't be resolved with a few extra hugs, a little more attention and some soft, tender words of understanding. For us, the trick has been to invest additional time and energy and appreciate Sarah has it tough too. Once we began to focus on her, she was able to handle the hard times with a lot more understanding and a little less "What about me?!"

———————————

CHAPTER 7

What About Me? —You, Your Spouse and Your Marriage

"I think it is cruel to expect the constant presence of any one family member. Just as we have to breathe in and breathe out, people have to 'recharge their batteries' outside the sickroom at times, live a normal life from time to time; we cannot function efficiently in the constant awareness of the illness. I have heard many relatives complain that members of the family went on pleasure trips over weekends or continued to go to a theater or movie. They blamed them for enjoying things while someone at home was terminally ill. I think it is more meaningful for the patient and his family to see that the illness does not totally disrupt a household or completely deprive all members of any pleasurable activities; rather, the illness may allow for a gradual adjustment and change toward the kind of home it is going to be when the patient is no longer around. Just as the terminally ill patient cannot face death all the time, the family member cannot and should not exclude all the other interactions for the sake of being with the patient exclusively. He too has a need to deny or avoid the sad realities at times in order to face them better when his presence is really needed."

—Dr. Elisabeth Kubler-Ross[1]

Journal Entry: June 1993

*We rely upon so many people for so many things. It seems
like all we do is take. I don't like the way this feels, but we
won't survive this if we don't take. I don't think it's possible
to do this on our own.*

*At work, I am forced to cancel meeting after meeting. I dis-
rupt the schedules of about fifty people per week, sometimes
more. I don't fear for my job because I work for a great company and a very good man, but at the same time I don't feel
like I'm doing my part. I can't finish anything. People have
begun to take me out of the loop because they can't rely on
me for results. I never know when I'm going to have to drop
everything and run. This is not good.*

Journal Entry: January 1994

*The roller coaster continues: several major victories besieged
by regular defeats. The only constant in our lives remains
the love and support we receive from family and friends—
gifts from God. Somehow we survive, but I now regularly
feel sorry for myself. This has been tougher than we could
have imagined. At times, it all seems so cruel. On reflection,
our family is growing stronger and closer. I have not yet sorted
it all out.*

Journal Entry: June 1994

*I don't think I can balance this anymore. How can I possibly
be a good father, husband, caregiver, boss and employee? I
don't seem to make anybody happy, and I'm too tired to
care, which bothers me more than anything. People depend
on me at home and at work. I'm responsible for the well-
being of so many people. At this point, I'm not sure if I can
even get from my bed to the bathroom without falling down.
How can I be responsible for more than myself in this condition?*

Journal Entry: May 1995

This is slowly killing Deborah. She bears the brunt of the daily misery. At least I get away to work. She watches our daughter's slow deterioration almost every minute of every day. It becomes numbing.

Though the tumors are growing inside of Amanda, they are consuming Deborah just as quickly. I can see her spirit being eaten away piece by piece. Pain for Amanda is pain for Deborah.

I arrive at the hospital tonight to find her staring out the window, which merely faces another part of the building and more hospital rooms filled with other children who are defined in terms of this or that disease. But she doesn't see the buildings or the people; she's deep within herself.

In her eyes, I can see that she longs for another day. I know that she thinks about the time before we were married, when children were a fantasy and obligations were few. Her dream was to live on a beach in Florida, with her kids at her side running down the sand towards the water. She'd teach them to surf and they'd live carefree lives. The call for sunshine and good waves would be the greatest concerns of the day. Instead, today she resides on the south side of Chicago, in a hospital room watching her daughter fight for her life. She never sees the sun. She's in Amanda's room before the sun comes up and leaves long after it sets. She and her daughter are anything but carefree. Rather than running together towards the ocean, it's all Deborah can do to get Amanda out of bed and to the bathroom; they take small, inchworm steps with three IV infusion pumps rolling behind them in tow.

This is not what she expected, and it eats her up inside. Deborah is one who needs to dream. She has always lived in terms of what the future might hold rather than what the world has to offer her today. But in our reality there is no future. We take life five minutes at a time. To dream is only to find disappointment. To plan is only to busy our minds and distract us from what lays ahead. Our plans are never realized, even those we make for the very next day.

So now my wife sits before me, but her mind drifts off to a time when I was not a part of her life; a time when she pictured me and her children to have turned out so differently. To really see me tonight is only to be reminded of just how shattered her dreams have become. To really deal with me tonight is only to deal with a painful present circumstance. We greet each other with a smile, but we'll not have any real conversation. We'll deal with what we have to, but only with what we have to. There'll be no honesty tonight or tomorrow, or the day after that.

And so we handle our pain separately, differently. Our lives move in different directions, though we sit in the same room, dealing with the same sad situation. We speak, but we hear each other as though in a dream—not really sure what the other person has said, or what it means. We listen, but only to the extent that it meets our most immediate needs.

I watch as Deborah kisses Amanda goodnight. We kiss each other as well, but there is no passion or longing in our lips; it's merely what we're supposed to do. Deborah leaves the room and Amanda and I pause for a moment. We've done this transition so many times before, but we need time to make the break.

I settle into the room. I'll be here for the next three days. Deborah drives home. And so it goes.

What About Me?—You, Your Spouse and Your Marriage

As parents, we put our needs behind those of our children. As caregivers we put the patient first. As sons and daughters, we try not to burden our parents and siblings with too much of the sorrow. As husbands and wives, we slowly become another member of the team—the other person to help accomplish all of the above.

There is no time for intimacy and no peace with which to want it. Our identities soon become intertwined with activities aimed at survival, not growth. I am no longer husband, I am provider of health insurance and weekend caregiver. I am no longer friend and lover, I am father and mother to "the healthy child" who still lives at home. We all become something other than what we had imagined.

Chaos turns into painful routine. We get used to the midnight runs to the hospital. We get used to the bad news. We get used to the obligatory weeks in the hospital. We get used to disappointment. We get used to canceled plans. We get used to being apart. We get used to the boredom, mixed with moments of high anxiety.

In order to shut out the pain, we don't allow ourselves happiness. To feel joy would make us vulnerable to misery. Even as one of us feels pain, it is often difficult to console the other because we are protecting our own inner selves. We have no strength to prop up our spouse, it's all reserved for ourselves or for our children. In fact, to show anything other than numbness almost becomes a sign of weakness, an annoyance.

We begin to find it almost strange to be alone together. The occasional intimate moment seems awkward now, almost forced. As a result, none of our spousal, parental or individual needs is met. It leaves us asking the question, "What about me?"

The Marriage

Sooner or later, almost every marriage comes to an impasse of sorts—a battle between individual egos, regardless of circumstances. It may take weeks or it may take years, but it almost always happens. While the thought of becoming a couple at first seems tantalizing and exciting, the novelty begins to wear off. Before long, some people feel trapped and suppressed, wondering why they got into this relationship in the first place. Husbands and wives often struggle to understand and maintain their own identify amidst the constant pressure to think and act like the "other half" of the duo.

The long-term success of a marriage typically depends upon each spouse's ability to keep his or her own ego in check, while at the same time valuing individual differences. When this occurs, each partner ultimately feels free to express him or herself as an individual but also sees how the spouse complements his or her strengths. When this stage is reached, relationships flourish. Husbands and wives value each other's contributions, but they also find joy in individuality—both their own and that of their spouse.

But what happens when trauma is introduced into the mix? What happens when your child's illness becomes larger than anything else around you? Do you and your spouse come closer together, or do you separate further? Do you put all the petty differences between you aside and see only the good, or do the differences become all that much more divisive? Do you become more reliant on your partner, or do you sink deep within yourself to find strength?

Any number of responses are possible, and you may react with any one of them depending on what stage you're at in marriage and how serious your child's condition is at the time. Deborah and I have reacted in many different ways over the past five years, including all the scenarios I mentioned above. We have been on the absolute brink of divorce (twice) and we have soared to tremendous highs when we made it through tough times together. But mostly, we tolerated each other's differences because we were unable to care for Amanda apart. We learned divorce was not an option, and we struggled to make it through our lives intact as husband and wife.

Deborah and I are very different people. Deborah is outgoing, while I am reserved. Deborah is often pessimistic, while I am more optimistic. Deborah fantasizes about the future, while I am grounded in the present. Deborah is influenced by things like weather and location, while I am more influenced by the way I feel inside. Deborah views Amanda's illness with bitterness, while I seek to find a way to live with hope.

To an impartial observer, we seem perfect for each other. Deborah opens me up, while I help her stay a little more focused. Deborah helps me stay more in touch with sensory experiences, while I help her find more of her inner self. Deborah helps me to dream, while I help her to find more happiness in our life today. Deborah helps me to understand Amanda's pain, while I help her to see Amanda as more than just a body ravaged by illness. *We complement each other perfectly.*

In the pressure cooker of Amanda's illness, however, we could hardly see these complementary qualities about each other. To see value in diverse perspectives requires time and thought, whereas all our interaction was forced into brief, stress-filled encounters as we changed shifts at the hospital or at home. When important, life-changing decisions need to be made quickly, differences only seem to get in the way, they become divisive and cause pain. And since we already had enough pain in our lives, we chose to avoid the anguish between us. In short, we stopped communicating with each other, and we stopped growing together.

Amanda's illness became our life. All our activities already centered around her care, but we also allowed it to define who we were as people. It became our only common bond. It became the thing for which we stood. We became "the couple with the sick little girl." People would marvel at our ability to stay together in spite of the illness. In fact, the illness was the only thing keeping us together at all!

Our toughest times came when Amanda entered a relatively healthy phase and things returned to a somewhat normal life. It was then our common bond broke and we had to face each other as individuals and as a couple. It was then we had the time to consider our own personal egos. It was then we felt the deepest void between us. It was also then we realized how little was left for each of us individually.

Deborah felt trapped at home since she couldn't even consider taking a job because Amanda often required all-day care. She hated life in the North, especially the cold weather, and felt removed from her family in Florida. While I could at least get away to work, Deborah lived Amanda's illness full time. She had no escape from the constant reminders of Amanda's pain, and her anxiety seemed to be all she had to claim as her own. Her stress would come out in explosive displays of extreme behavior, which I viewed as childish and outrageous.

I, on the other hand, felt I was not pleasing anybody. I was too stressed to be worth much at work, my wife was unhappy, my healthy daughter was ignored and Amanda's life seemed to be hanging by a thread. I felt like a failure and often went deep within myself, dealing only at the surface level with anyone I encountered, including my own wife. This, in turn, made Deborah feel ignored. She became despondent over my lack of understanding, which only made me want to be further away from her, and of course that made Deborah feel even worse.

But just as things would start to come to a boiling point between us, Amanda would get sick again and we kicked back into survival mode. We divided up tasks and conquered. Once again our minds were filled with concern over Amanda's condition, and we had no room for our differences. In fact, our common bond had returned and we could need each other again. It almost became easier to be together when Amanda was the sickest. It was a perverse paradigm that continued for years.

However, thanks to much prayer and the guidance of the Lord, we made it through that difficult period. Our love has blossomed and become stronger from our experience. Today we look to each other for support, friendship, intimacy and strength.

We find peace in each other's company and joy in togetherness. This is not to say we don't fall into the same traps every now and again; it merely means we are able to overcome them.

I would like to share with you several factors that led to this turnaround. Although many of these points are applicable if you are a single parent or if your children are perfectly healthy, for married couples with ill children, they may be critical to your long-term relationship.

Pointers to Save Your Marriage and/or Your Sanity

For Deborah and me, the key was to integrate Amanda's illness into the rest of our lives. For five years, her illness was our life; we had nothing else. We may have given the appearance of doing other things, but her illness dominated our every thought. We lived it perpetually inside our souls. Although we had done everything we could to help Amanda feel as normal and care-free as possible, we did not allow ourselves the same luxury. Our anxiety over her condition became more prevalent in every aspect of our lives until there was no more Scott, there was no more Deborah and there was no more "us."

After our marriage hit bottom, the time finally came when we knew we had to define ourselves and Amanda as something other than her sickness. We still had all the same problems, but we began to deal with them differently. We started looking at Amanda's illness as a part of our lives, not our life itself. We began to deal with problems as they occurred, not in anticipation of the next occurrence. We began to plan activities and follow through with them even if things weren't perfect with Amanda's health. *In short, we began to take back control of our lives.*

It wasn't easy to do. It often involved a lot of extra work to make things come together, even if we were tired and it would have been easier to get a couple of extra hours of sleep. It involved putting up with some raised eyebrows when people would question our plans to do things with Amanda so ill at home. And it involved accepting disappointment when our plans fell through because Amanda was just too sick. Still, it was better to have tried and failed than to allow ourselves to wallow in the misery.

The human psyche is interesting. People become comfortable with what they know, even if they know only pain and sorrow. Before long, it dominates their lives. As the saying goes, "you are what you think." If you think you're miserable, you will be. In fact, in a strange way you begin to feel better when you're miserable. You'll actually begin to subconsciously seek out misery. After all, it's what you know best. You know how to deal with it, even if it is unpleasant.

Perhaps the trick, then, is to not allow yourself to become comfortable with the pain. We must actively seek joy even in the midst of tragedy. As parents of seriously ill children, we must make a conscious effort to step out of the illness and see all that is still good around us. We must break the cycle that drags us down and allow ourselves to feel good about feeling good. That is not to say we won't feel pain and sorrow, but we will not let it rule our entire lives. We must look past the IV tubes and the dark, sullen eyes of our children and try to see the sparkling eyes of youth. Then we must look into our hearts and see the same thing.

As Deborah and I broke free, we were able to become individuals again. We could experience something other than sickness and feel OK about it. We no longer felt guilty about having some fun once in awhile, and we could allow ourselves to think of something other than our problems. While this amounts to much less time than the average family has to be carefree, it was enough to break us out of the five-year "spiral of sorrow."

As we felt more like normal people (at least closer to normal), Deborah and I were able to look for the love that brought us together in the first place. While this was very difficult at first (in fact, things got worse for a while), we began to recover from the destructive mode we had created. We allowed each other to be different and to celebrate those differences. We allowed each other the space necessary to be who we are and to see how that could complement our family life.

Today, we are able to enter the tough times with Amanda knowing we will be OK. After all, the tough times are part of our life too. It's just that now we define ourselves in terms of family and self first, and illness a distant second. *We integrate the tough times into our family life and not the family life into the tough times.* This is not a point of semantics; it's a critical point that can make the difference between joy and sorrow.

If you find yourself in the same position, let me encourage you to begin putting the illness into perspective with the rest of your life. It will not be easy, especially in the early years. Life-changing conditions often require a complete shift in one's perspective, which may have taken thirty years or more to develop. We can't be expected to turn it around overnight. But we must turn it around eventually for the sake of our children, our spouse and ourselves.

As you begin to break out of the mold you created for yourself, you may want to consider some of these other thoughts as well. Each of these points could help you identify either where you are in your relationship, or how you might want to approach the next step toward positive change:

- In order to grow together, both husband and wife must reach the "acceptance" phase of dealing with their child's illness. Until both partners can deal with their own feelings about the illness honestly and with acceptance, it will be difficult to deal with your feelings as a couple. As long as either the husband or the wife remains bitter or in denial, the marriage relationship will be filled with bitterness and denial.

- Part of this acceptance implies your life has changed. You face a potentially long and difficult road that will be unlike anything you may have pictured before or even after you got married. Things are different now. The challenge is to find the joy buried deep in your new circumstance.

- You must also accept there will be times when you can't be together. You may go weeks at a time when circumstances require you be apart from your spouse and children. You must be very aware this can be destructive to your relationship and resolve to make up for it when you are together.

- After the periods of separation, make sure you find the time to get away as a couple. This can be as simple as a special dinner at a restaurant close by the hospital while your child sleeps, or it may be a long weekend at a nearby hotel while someone qualified watches your children. You can still be home quickly if needed. If things are somewhat stable, get away completely.

- During your time away as a couple, allow yourselves some quiet time. Don't feel you have to solve all the problems of your relationship during dinner or over a weekend. Sometimes just being together in silence can bring you closer together than trying to tackle difficult issues. If you have the time or inclination to communicate, great—but don't force it.

- Try not to tackle important issues when you're both tired or in the middle of a critical decision. Stress and tension will be high at these times. Also, don't feel the need to resolve all of your issues at once. Take one or two at a time and work on those for a while. Be patient. Your marriage is worth it.

- Make sure you allow yourself some time by yourself. Although being out of the house running errands is at least a break from the hospital or home care, it is still activity aimed at family care. Each spouse should arrange some time for the other to get away and focus on him or herself for awhile without any obligation to others. This time away, focused 100 percent on yourself, will give you needed time to reconcile personal feelings, both about the illness and other aspects of your life.

- Whenever you have the chance, take time to *love* your spouse. Work at it. Hold hands, bring home flowers, rub your partner's back. Say "I love you" or "I couldn't live without your" now and then. There is rarely a "convenient" time in this situation to be loving, but you must make the time. These moments are *critical* to you now.

- Read the book *I Will Never Leave You* by Gayle and Hugh Prather. Although it gets into some unnecessary and strange areas at times, it also teaches you how to find what's good in your partner. It shows you the futility in leaving your spouse and the way to work through relationship problems. This book was incredibly important to me and I've read it twice. I highly recommend it.

- In the midst of all the stress, devote some energy to your own health. If possible, sleep outside of the hospital room on occasion, exercise at least once or twice a week and eat right. This will both reduce stress and make you physically more prepared to handle the all-nighters.

Although much of this chapter may sound incredibly selfish, it is not. If you do not do these things, you could be heading toward a path of personal destruction that will ultimately make life more difficult for your child. Think about it. If your marriage falls apart, will that help your child's healing? If you run yourself into the ground, will you be able to care for your child when you also get sick? If you begin to define yourself only in terms of their illness, might they not also begin to define themselves only in terms of their illness? And if you cannot find joy in your life anymore, how can you show your child how to find it?

Your parental instincts will work against you as you try to find time for yourself and each other. They will tell you never to leave your child's side. They will tell you to put your own needs aside for the needs of your child. And much of the time, these instincts are right on track. But if the illness drags on over months or years, you must begin to integrate your child's needs into the needs of the family, the needs of the marriage and your needs as a child of God.

It is my strong belief if we do these things, we make life much better for our children and every other member of the family. By becoming a joyful person, you show your children joy. By becoming a loving spouse, you support your life partner through an incredibly difficult time in his or her life. And by allowing yourself to grow, you begin to realize the potential God has in store for you.

If we plant despair, we will harvest only despair. If we expect misery, we will find only misery. But if we plant seeds of love and happiness, we will harvest love, happiness, strength and peace. Along the way, we will be amazed at how our view of the world has changed.

---

1. Adapted with the permission of Simon & Schuster from *On Death and Dying* by Elisabeth Kubler-Ross. Copyright © 1969 by Elisabeth Kubler-Ross.

CHAPTER 8

What About Me?
—Family and Friends

*"Ever since Amanda became ill, I have read
countless books on death, dying and chronic
illness . . . all in a vain search for something
that would tell me exactly what to say, how
I should act, what I should do, when I
should do it and how I should feel. Needless
to say, I now know that I never will find
such a book. How we relate to those that we
love comes from the heart, and it is there
that I now search for what to say to you."*

—Sherry (MacLellan) Linkous

A Letter to My Parents: October 1993

Dear Mom and Dad,

*I know you are both somewhat apprehensive about the up-
coming living donor transplant and how I will fare, so I
thought I'd take a few moments to share my thoughts with
you.*

*First let me say that I understand your concern. You care for
me and Sherry as much as I care for Sarah and Amanda.
You naturally worry about my well-being as much as I worry
about the well-being of my children. I appreciate your anxi-*

ety over my future. But just as you think of my future, I must think about the future of my children. Amanda faces a very tough road ahead and we must all do what is required to give her the same chance that we have had in life.

I also realize that you share a concern for Deborah and Sarah if something should happen to me. Believe me, I have agonized over this. At this point, however, we are talking about survival. Individuals and families make tough choices when survival is at stake. This is my—and our—tough choice. The decision is made. Now is the time to move forward and ensure the best possible outcome for our Amanda. Second-guessing will only add to the difficulty of the situation.

Most important, however, you need to know that throughout all of this—past, present and future—I go forth without fear, but rather with a deep sense of peace, a certainty that no matter what happens, the Will of God will triumph—triumph over all the problems that seem to over-shadow us at this point in time.

I give of my body willingly and lovingly, not only because Amanda is my daughter, but because my body is such a small part of who I am. I define myself in a way that is far more vast than what my frame would show. I am a spirit that extends itself through the love of Christ. I am a spirit that is joined with you and all our brothers in Christ. Together, we make up the Son of God. Together, we will put aside our bodies and this world and return to a place that is far more joyous than we can imagine. How could I fear anything when such a glorious outcome is so certain?! Put your faith in this and you will find a similar peace.

Now, what if something should happen to me? Well, I'd ask that you do the following:

—Take care of Deborah, Sarah and (hopefully) Amanda.

—*Grieve for me if that is what you feel. But grieve with a sense of hope, hope that I am still very much alive, hope that I am still with you in your hearts and minds.*

—*Hold no grievances, no regrets. I will have done what was required and done it without hesitation. Turn and look for me. I will be there with you.*

All of this will, of course, seem very silly in about a month when we are all doing fine, much as all fears and concerns ultimately seem distant and unimportant once we have overcome whatever obstacle seemed to be before us. I'll look forward to that time when we can look back favorably on the choices we have made.

I hope this helps you to understand and accept the decision I have made. Most of all, I hope that you find peace in all of life's circumstance. Only those choices that bring peace to your spirit are the choices that match the Will of God. This decision has brought peace to mine.

Peace and love be with you all the days of your lives.

Excerpts from a letter from my sister: March 1996

". . . I remember hearing from Mom and Dad that Amanda was near the end. I had prayed for so long that things would get better for you, but I realized now that all my hopes of wellness and normalcy for your family were shattered. I went into the dining room and started throwing things as hard as I could against the wall. I was so mad I could not speak. Bob came in and had to pin me down so I would stop. He just held me and I cried my heart out. I have never in my life cried so hard as that night. It was like all the anger that I had stored up over the past three years was pouring out of my body. It no longer consumed me.

I don't understand why this has had to happen to you, but I guess I accept that it has now. I don't blame anyone for it anymore. I don't feel guilty for having healthy children, nor do I feel that I'm not allowed to feel frustrated once in a while with things that occur in my own life! When and if Amanda leaves us, it will be more than any of us can bear, most of all you, Deborah and Sarah. But I know we need to focus on the good things right now, and one way or another we all will come out on the other side. I also feel that you must know how much I care for you and that you can count on me, just like I know I can always count on you . . ."

What About Me?—Family and Friends

I was talking with a friend at work the other day and he was very upset about the booster shot his son had gotten the day before. The shot was traumatizing for his child, but what made matters worse was my friend had to be at work and couldn't be with his son during his ordeal. He went on for about ten minutes, talking about how anguished both he and his son were over this "incident." Then he asked about Amanda.

What was I supposed to say? "Well, this morning she got up and took more medicine than your son will ever take in his lifetime. Right now she's in the hospital (while I'm here at work) getting a needle stuck in her chest to access a catheter that goes directly into her heart. They're pumping three different poisons into her system that will make her feel horrible for the next two weeks. During that time, she'll swell up like a balloon and have migraine headaches. Afterwards, she'll go down to radiology where they'll pump two different chemicals into her bloodstream that burn like fire so they can give her a CT scan. Then if we're lucky, she won't get sick while her immune system is down and end up back in the hospital" (which did happen three days later).

Of course, that's not what I said. He loves Amanda and he asked out of genuine concern for her well-being. But to respond truthfully as to what's happening in our lives—even to friends who care about us—literally leaves them speechless. They feel awkward for having asked about an obviously painful subject and they have no point of reference with which to respond. They're blown away by the realities of what we're dealing with and not sure if they should dig deeper to show their concern, or let it go out of respect for our privacy. Your silence only adds to their discomfort and they struggle to find a way out of the conversation.

Sometimes even family members don't know what to say or do. In our case, they ache for us and Amanda, but they aren't sure when to be actively supportive or quietly understanding. For example, even though my sister and I are very close, she was uncertain as to what she should do to support our family through the early stages of Amanda's illness. She wanted to come to Chicago to see Amanda and help us (she lives near Baltimore), but she was worried coordinating the trip with our many unscheduled, lengthy trips to the hospital would make her visit more of a burden than a help. She wanted to call us but didn't want us to have to describe Amanda's condition for the hundredth time. And she wanted to let me know how much pain she too was feeling but didn't want to "complain" when we had so much on our minds.

For years, she was hesitant to share the problems she was experiencing in her own life, thinking they were minor in comparison to Amanda's situation. My parents would do the same thing and so would our very close friends. But what happened along the way is we all stopped communicating. Amanda's illness seemed to be the only thing people thought was "worth" talking about, but they were often uncomfortable with how to talk about it. The end result was nobody around us really talked at all.

At the same time, Deborah and I struggled to communicate our feelings and needs to those around us. Many times, the pain was too deep for words. Other times, *we* weren't sure what was happening with Amanda, making it difficult to describe the situation to our friends or to our families who live a thousand miles away. We were completely confused and our frustration sometimes came out as anger, making those who asked about Amanda unsure if they should ever ask again. Often, we were just too tired and/or depressed to recap the events of the day and would avoid conversation all together. Talking about the illness was the last thing we wanted to do. We wanted quiet time to sort it all out, or just to feel bad about it—by ourselves.

As a result, we gradually became distant from family and friends. We got tired of making all the phone calls required to keep everyone up-to-date. We got tired of talking about pain and suffering all the time. We also just got tired—flat out physically exhausted. Sleep became more important than interaction. Social activity became frivolous or impossible due to Amanda's condition. In short, we became isolated from the very network of people who could have helped us the most.

Along the way, our family and friends felt like they were not only losing Amanda, they were losing us. They became caught in a no-win situation where they wanted to show support, but they did not want to intrude. They wanted to know about Amanda but not become a burden. They wanted to actively participate in this very important part of our lives but were being pushed away by they very people they were looking to help. It left them asking, "What about me!?"

Involving Family and Friends

As Deborah and I began to integrate Amanda's illness into our lives, we became aware of how the people around us were feeling about her illness as well. But not all of this increased awareness came through personal insight. Our friends and family members had to share their feelings with us.

I realized this when I recently went through a program at work that allowed people in my department to give me confidential feedback on my performance as a manager. I received input from about fifteen direct reports, my peers and my boss.

When I got the report back, I was amazed to find what they wanted to talk about was not so much about how I manage them, or what was going on with our business but rather what was happening with Amanda. After five years of walking on egg-shells around the subject, they had finally found a communication vehicle that allowed them to talk about her ill-ness without threat of feeling embarrassed or uncomfortable.

Over the years, each of them would occasionally ask how she was doing and I would give them my standard responses to avoid putting them, or me, on the spot. But now they wanted to know what was really going on and how they could talk about it in the future without being afraid to ask. They wanted to let me know how they really felt about what we were going through and how hurtful it was to them too. They wanted me to feel I could trust them to share some of the pain. They wanted to know maybe they could make a mistake and say something "stu-pid" in an effort to better communicate with me.

Incredibly, within the same week I received a six-page let-ter from my sister. She had written me many supportive notes over the years, but this note was about how *she* felt about every-thing. It was about her deep hurt over seeing Amanda's physical pain and my emotional pain. It was about how she took her anger out on her own family and on God. It was about how she wouldn't allow herself or her own daughters to complain about anything, since "they were healthy and had it so much better than Amanda." It was about her difficult search to understand why this happened to Amanda, to me, to Deborah and to Sarah. It was about how she finally came to grips with the reality of Amanda's illness and how she finally reconciled her feelings.

This time it was my turn to be blown away and speechless. Just as other people had no point of reference for what Deborah and I were feeling, I had none for what they had been feeling. I was so caught up in my emotions I had become numb to those around me. I finally realized those who love and care for our family were struggling too.

They too were trying to understand why this happened to Amanda. They too were trying to integrate her illness into their lives. They wanted to care for Amanda, but didn't have the benefit of being with her to tend to her needs and soothe her spirit. Their need to nurture her was left unfulfilled; all that was left was the anguish of wondering how she was doing each and every moment. Their desire to nurture Deborah and me also was left unfulfilled, leaving them feeling as though they were no support at all. It wasn't an easy journey for them either.

Supporting Each Other

Now that I've learned more about how people around me feel and what their needs are, I have attempted to be more open about Amanda. I've attempted to let them see how we have integrated her illness into our lives and let them share in the joy of how well she is doing with her treatment. This has been tough for me as I am a very private person. It's also been awkward at times for all of us, but I hope I can find the balance between what I am comfortable with sharing and what needs to be shared.

Still, I'm sure many questions remain for those family members and friends of parents with seriously ill children who are reading this book and wondering how they can talk to and support their loved ones. What follows are some thoughts on how to reach out to your family or friends in their time of need so you can stay connected and nurture each other through a very difficult time. I've based these thoughts on our experiences with wonderful friends, loving family members and thoughtful "strangers" who were a very important part of our lives over the past several years. I hope some of these ideas might work for you.

Communicating With the Parents About the Illness

Communicating with parents about their child's illness can be difficult, not only because it's a sensitive topic but because each parent handles the subject differently. For instance, I don't like to talk much about Amanda's condition at all. Deborah, on the other hand, usually finds it therapeutic to talk about Amanda and might even bring up the situation to complete strangers. For both of us, however, our readiness to discuss Amanda's condition may vary depending on how well Amanda is feeling at the time and her current prognosis.

You might find people are more willing to talk about their children as they become more successful at integrating the illness into their everyday lives. As I think about my experience, I realize in the early stages of Amanda's illness I wasn't ready to talk about it outside of my family and circle of very close friends. I was on an emotional roller coaster and had no idea what I was really feeling or what Amanda was really going through. Since I did not understand my own feelings and since the "wound" was still fresh, it was very difficult and painful to discuss Amanda with other people.

As time went by, I was able to communicate what was happening and how I was feeling, but I was also looking to escape from her illness once in awhile. I thought about her almost every second of every day and talking about it all the time only served to deepen my discomfort. Eventually I became hungry for conversation that would force me to think about things outside of her condition.

Today I am able to talk about it without reservation, but I do not want to be the one to bring it up. I'd rather not make her illness the topic of conversation, but I'm also very willing to help others understand what's happening if they want to know. However, I still struggle with how to put it into perspective so people aren't blown away in the process. Talking about her prognosis, for example, is difficult to do. People want to be reassured she'll be fine forever, but we're never sure from one month to the next exactly what her condition will be. When I mention that, some people become extremely uncomfortable.

Following are some thoughts on how you can communicate with the parents of an ill child to keep up-to-date and to show your support.

- In many cases, the most immediate communication need is for family and friends to get up-to-date information on the child's condition, since it can often change from one minute to the next. But making all the phone calls required to keep people informed can become burdensome for the parents, or stressful if the news is unclear or not good. How does one solicit information from the parents without creating problems in the process?

  You might recommend creating a phone chain, which is how we handle Amanda's updates. When we receive an update, we call one person in our family and they call the rest of the family. You can do the same thing at work or with friends. This will limit the amount of calls the parent needs to make, as well as allow them to update you when they are ready to talk about it.

- Sometimes things get very hectic and the parents of the child are unable to call with regular updates. Those without updated news may become anxious and try to track down the parents either at home or in the child's hospital room. But try to keep these calls to a minimum. The parents may be catching their only moments of sleep for the day (even if it's midafternoon), or they might be in the middle of an important medical procedure.

- Many people outside of the family or phone network want to know how they can show their support and inquire about the child without feeling as though they're being intrusive. In this case, you may consider sending a note or card to let the parents know how much you care. No need to be wordy if that's not what you're comfortable with; just a short note will send the message you're looking to convey. We've received many such cards and find it very uplifting to know how many people love us and Amanda.

- If you have really strong feelings about what's happening, go ahead and write a letter to the parents about how you're feeling. Let the parents know you want to support them any way you can. You also might say you'd like to talk more about it if they're ready to do so. This gives parents the option to respond to your request or to let it pass if they're not ready.

- Even if you are close to the parents, you might still consider sending a letter to express your support and perhaps even share your deepest feelings. Sometimes it's easier to write what you're feeling than to speak the words. Writing will give you time to think about how you really feel, as well as the time to choose the proper words to express those feelings.

A letter will also allow the parents of the child time to absorb and understand those feelings without feeling the pressure to respond to them one way or another. But whether you speak the words or write them, be sure to express them some way, somehow. I wish my sister had written her letter to me five years ago. I love her dearly and never wanted her to feel such pain alone. Perhaps we could have worked through it together instead of separately.

- If you want to probe for more information about the child, be prepared to handle some disquieting news or intense conversation. You might ask a question at the very moment the parent needs to talk and he or she will unload on you. So don't ask if you don't really want to know.

- If the parent does open up and you notice he or she is in denial or angry, don't try to change that. Just understand their position. Denial may be the parents only coping mechanism at the time, or they may need to feel anger in order to move on to another stage. You may even let them know you feel angry and confused about it too.

- Don't always feel the need to have answers for the parents. Most of the time they're not looking for answers, just somebody to talk to. In fact, there are times when answers will only shut them down because they're not ready to hear them yet. Sometimes quiet understanding and unconditional love is the best possible support you can offer.

- Don't be afraid to share things that are happening in your own life, even if they seem trivial in comparison. Any communication is good communication, so long as you don't come across as complaining. I shared with you earlier in this chapter the story of my friend with the son who got the booster shot. I was delighted he told me that story because it was very important to him and therefore it was important to me. It allowed us to continue our friendship in spite of Amanda's illness.

- Don't give up on the parents if they have rebuffed your offers of help. Gently remind them through brief comments or supportive notes that you are there for them. It took me five years to open up. A lot of people tried to crack my shell during that time, and it was only their *gentle* persistence that helped get me to where I am today—and I've still got a long way to go.

Helping Out

I can't begin to quantify all the different ways people have helped us over the years. Their response to our needs has been overwhelming, and completely necessary to our survival. We never would have made it through this without their help.

During the early stages of Amanda's illness many people struggled with how to help us; however; we didn't even know what we needed, let alone felt comfortable asking for anything. Thus you may find you need to ask a few probing questions to find the best way to support them. Here are some ideas you might consider when looking to be helpful.

- Taking care of the siblings is probably the greatest gift you can offer parents when a child is in the hospital. When Amanda's condition begins to worsen, knowing Sarah is in a safe, loving and carefree environment puts my mind at ease more than anything else. By having this burden removed from our minds, Deborah and I are free to concentrate on Amanda's needs, which can be all-consuming when she's not well.

There have been many times when our parents flew into Chicago just to take care of Sarah during lengthy hospital visits. Neighbors met Sarah at the school bus when a routine hospital visit turned into a twelve hour ordeal. These same neighbors took Sarah into their homes at one or two in the morning as we rushed Amanda off to the emergency room. Friends took Sarah and our dog for days or weeks at a time when things got really bad; and they drove her the four-hour round trip to visit her sister.

I cannot even begin to describe the intense love I feel even as I write these words, just thinking about how these people have cared for us by caring for Sarah. The impact of their efforts has been far greater than they will ever know.

- Perhaps the second greatest gift is baby-sitting so the parents can get away for dinner, a movie or a vacation on their own. When Amanda stabilizes, Deborah and I will do whatever we can to get away for a few days so we can renew our relationship. One neighborhood family even took our kids for ten days so Deborah could join me on a business trip out of the country. This was the first real quality time we had together in over a year.

This "marriage maintenance" is critical to the parents. While most couples have some time on their own every now and again, these mini-vacations or dinner dates may be the only quality time the couple has had in months. Sometimes even an hour or two alone will be enough to sustain them for another few months.

- If the parents of the child live far away from you but you still want to actively support them, write them a letter and ask if they wouldn't mind if you flew in to see them. If you're worried about becoming a burden in the process, tell them you'll rent a car and a hotel room. Let the parents know it is not their responsibility to entertain, cook or keep a clean house for you. In fact, perhaps you'd like to do all those things for them. Let them know you are there to see the child and support them and that is all you need, even if it means you don't see them much during your visit.

- Another way to support the parents is to consider the everyday chores left undone when the child is in the hospital. People have watered and mowed our lawn, put out the trash, shopped for groceries, cooked our meals, walked and fed our dog, picked up the mail and done many other helpful deeds. It's important to note however, several times they did these things without asking us. Had they asked, we would have felt very uncomfortable about imposing on them and would have said no.

One of my favorite stories about "quietly" helping out involves a very good friend of the family who works with me. Almost every day, he comes into my office and asks if there's anything he can do. He occasionally covers for me at work in my absence and his family often takes care of Sarah during lengthy hospital visits. But usually I thank him and say no.

One particular morning, however, he walked in and I was on my third day without sleep. As usual, he asked if he could do anything to help and I sarcastically said, "Yeah, you could shovel my driveway." We had been through a rough winter and had just gotten another foot of snow. I just didn't have the energy to shovel it again and since Amanda was already in the hospital, I had no immediate need to clear it.

He knew I was only kidding, so we laughed at my comment, talked awhile about business and each went about our day. But when I got up the next morning, my driveway was clear. Incredibly, he and his family had driven the half hour it takes to get to my house and in the dark of night (we live in the country and it gets very dark) removed all the snow. I was asleep and never even knew they were there. Although a clear driveway was a big help, the boost to my spirit did far more good than just enabling me to get out of the garage. This happened almost two years ago, but it still lifts my spirit to think about it.

- I believe, without question, prayer dramatically and positively impacts the outcome of an illness. I believe prayer is the reason Amanda is still here today. *Prayer will help the family*. You do not, however, need to tell the family you're praying for them. Prayer will have an effect with or without their knowledge. The beautiful thing about it is you can pray often and do it without ever having to approach the parents.

The Work Environment

If you are fortunate to have a supportive work environment, it can mean the difference between coping with the illness or cracking under its pressures. When a child is seriously ill, income and health insurance take on a whole new level of importance, and thus work-related issues can become very stressful. Parents not only have the pressures at work any job creates, but they have more pressure at home than anyone can understand.

I happen to have the most supportive work environment for which anyone could hope. When Amanda gets sick, my boss supports me without fail. Whatever I need, I get. If I need time off, I get it. If I need to miss an important meeting, that's OK. If I can't meet a deadline, he extends it. If I need to talk, he listens.

At the same time, my peers and direct reports cover for me whenever Amanda ends up in the hospital. They do much of my work while I'm out and limit their contact with me to allow me to concentrate on Amanda. When I return to the office, they bring me back up to speed and give me time to ease back into the daily routine.

Yet despite all this support, I had anxiety over my work situation in the first few years of Amanda's illness. I worried I wasn't pulling my weight or I was holding people back. I was forever messing up my co-workers' schedules because I'd have to leave work in a rush to be with Amanda at the hospital.

It became very difficult to manage my job, which was our only source of income and health insurance. Although I never felt I would lose my position because of my absence, I felt as though I was slowly being left out of the loop, rendering me ineffective in the long run. I also just felt bad I wasn't doing my part.

At one point, I was working weekends to catch up. During the week I'd be at my desk by 5 A.M. and not leave until 7 P.M. I also ended up traveling as much as five days a week when Amanda was well, since that was a big part of my job. I had no downtime. When I wasn't under the pressure of Amanda's illness, I was under self-imposed pressure at work.

The result, of course, was burnout and anxiety, which left me worn out and susceptible to illness. Since I was almost always around sick people in the hospital, I was almost always getting sick, which added even more stress. Had I not had such a supportive environment at work, I truly might have cracked.

For those of you who work with people in my situation, there are some important ways in which you can be supportive:

- Apply all the same principles already mentioned in the "help-ing out" and "communications" sections in this chapter. Communications, in particular, may be strained since some work environments do not allow for personal interaction. Sending a supportive note may be the best option in that case.

- Be supportive and completely flexible with schedules, no matter what the needs of the business are at the time.

- Never make the person feel guilty about what he or she missed or didn't accomplish. The person probably already feels guilty and anxious about it.

- If the employee requests it, you can keep them up to speed on work issues by sending phone mails, memos or mail clearly separated into urgent, moderately-urgent or not-urgent cat-egories. This will keep the person current and able to handle only the most urgent issues—or nothing at all—when things are at their worst.

Hospital stays often include long waiting periods, leading to intense boredom. I would often do my phone and regular mail when Amanda napped and be thankful I had some-thing to do during this time. By keeping current with work-related issues while I was out, I was better prepared when I returned to the office, making for a less stressful tran-sition.

- If you're the parent's boss or in human resources, find out if the health insurance is working out. Run interference for your employee if the insurance company is inappropriately giving him or her a hard time. This could be a critical.

- The boss should send supportive messages, written or ver-bal, to the employee. He or she may have a critical need to know of your support, even though he or she isn't produc-ing for the company at that particular time. Let your employee know you're along for the long haul and you know he or she will be back again when possible. Bosses will find they have the most loyal employee ever once he or she is back.

- Be alert to burnout. Self-motivated employees will push themselves to extreme. Although you want to let them work hard if they have a need to (as I did), don't let them push themselves too far.

What Can the Parents of the Child Do?

As parents of ill children, we also have obligations. We need to be sensitive to the needs of others who are concerned about our child's illness. Here are some thoughts as to how you can be supportive to those around you without pushing yourself over the edge:

- Be aware family members in particular have a need know how things are going with the child. Don't be frustrated with them for asking questions, especially if they don't live near you and do not have direct access to the child.

- Call your phone chain contacts as often as you can to keep information current. Even a sixty-second phone conversation can ease a day's worth of anxiety for many people who are worried about the child and you.

- If you're ready to talk about the illness at all, share your feelings with your parents and siblings. They are dying inside for you and want to be there for you. Let them be your outlet. Don't feel the need to protect them from your problem. They would rather be protecting you.

- Every once in awhile, ask your family members how they're doing or how they're feeling about the whole thing. They may be looking desperately for a way to talk to you but are afraid to do so. Give them a sign that it's OK to talk.

- Accept help. People want to help and feel better having done so. I denied this help for years and it made life more difficult for our family, and harder for people to communicate with me.

We all have needs, regardless of our circumstance in life. But when a child becomes seriously ill, there seems to be a special pain we all feel, creating a unique set of needs that cry out for attention. Along the way, we can only make it to the end of our journey if we help and support each other. The parents of the child clearly won't make it without assistance, and those who love and care for them won't fare as well without connecting with the parents. It's in this coming together the greatest peace is found.

CHAPTER 9

Where Is God
in All This?

*"Sometimes, God doesn't change
our circumstances, he changes us
in our circumstances."*
—Carla Killough McClafferty[1]

Journal Entry: August 1991

*Amanda runs fevers almost every night, so midnight trips to
the hospital have become commonplace. We go to bed each
night wondering not if the fever will come, but when it will
come. Sometimes I just lay awake in bed waiting for Sarah
to let us know that Amanda needs help. It seems easier to
stay up through the night than to go to sleep in the first place.
I have come to dread the sound of my name being called out
from the darkness.*

*Last night was the worst yet. After waking to the sound of a
more urgent call than usual, Deborah and I leaped from the
bed and ran upstairs. When we got to the girls' room, Sarah
had Amanda in her arms, telling her that everything would
be OK. Amanda was shivering so hard she was almost con-
vulsing. While we usually wait to see if we can get the fever
to break, this time I got her right into the car and took her to
the hospital.*

Six hours later we were sitting on the same hospital stretcher that had served as "home base" all night and Amanda had fallen asleep in my arms. She had the IV antibiotics running through the line that had taken four attempts and two hours to get started. The IV is always the worst part because her veins collapse every time an attempt is made to start one. I don't know how Deborah deals with this so often.

I was exhausted and numb. Too tired to be aware of much of anything, I stared at my child for at least an hour. And then for the first time I asked myself, Why? Why Amanda? Why our family? Why me?! I had avoided those questions for months, but now they came flooding through my mind at light speed. It was almost as though all my built-up emotions were being crushed into this very moment with these very questions.

And suddenly I remembered back to a sermon I'd heard a few years before. The Pastor told the story of a girl who had been in a car accident and had glass in her eyes. The child's father had to hold his daughter down while the doctors pulled out the glass, which was very painful for her. The girl cried out, "Daddy, why are you hurting me?" The father was crushed, but continued his task because he knew it was the right thing for his daughter.

I thought of this, not in the context of what I was doing for Amanda, but what the Lord was doing for me. And then suddenly, I sensed very strongly that Christ was right there in the room with me; suffering for me as passionately as I was suffering for Amanda. I swear He was right in that examining room with me, comforting me. I couldn't see Him, but He was there. And as I felt His presence, my rage turned to peace. I gave Amanda over to God. His will be done.

Two hours later, we were given the clearance to leave the ER and we returned home. Deborah and Sarah were having breakfast. I shaved, showered, dressed and went to work.

Journal Entry: February 1993

Things are getting worse. Amanda's liver is failing. Prognosis is not good. I feel helpless. I must turn it over to God.

Journal Entry: May 1993

Today I told Amanda that I want to be like her when I grow up. Her smile turned cold and she said, "No, Daddy, if you were me, then you'd be sick. You just be the Daddy."

Though the body is broken, her spirit is far healthier than mine.

Journal Entry: January 1994

I now look to the Bible and to prayer for answers—and do find them there. God and Christ are not of this world. We will not find them here in perfect bodies and perfect lives. Our challenge is to find them despite imperfection, despite the whims of the gods of this world. We must look beyond the ordinary, into the extraordinary to find peace in the midst of outright injustice and cruelty.

God, Christ and the Holy Spirit are always with me. It's my job to stop and listen for their voice.

Journal Entry: February 1994

I have spent much time in prayer and in quiet contemplation. I read everything I can find on God, spirituality and religion. There is still so much I do not understand, so much that conflicts and contradicts.

Still, there are some constants, some basic themes that repeat over and over and over again. These are the tenets that I now look to for a foundation. They have become the unchanging aspects of my ever-changing world. They are what I shall hold onto for the rest of my life, and life after life. For me they are keys to happiness:

1. Love God with all your heart, soul and mind.

2. Trust in Jesus Christ as your Lord and Savior.

3. Listen for the voice of the Holy Spirit. He is with you always, trying to lead you back to God.

4. Love your brother as yourself.

5. Forgive. Forgiveness is a requirement of love. It flows naturally from love. This will bring you peace more than any other component.

6. Know that another, more glorious life awaits you. No matter how unfair this life may seem, there are wonders beyond your current experience.

7. Cling not to this world. There is nothing here more important than God, Christ and the Holy Spirit, not your house, not your job, not your friends, not your family.

Nothing!

In many ways, this will be the easiest lesson I will ever learn; and in many ways, it will be the most difficult. It will always be the most important.

Journal Entry: December 1994

After a month of only minor problems, Amanda spiked a high fever again. It's amazing how this cycle goes. Just when you think you can settle back into a routine and plan out your life, a single call for help in the middle of the night changes everything. Within thirty seconds of the call, you realize that everything you had planned gets put on hold: career plans, vacations plans, holiday plans, business travel, day-to-day activities, etc. Within sixty seconds of the call, you're reminded that you don't have a normal life. You must live day to day because you are unable to do otherwise.

Perhaps that's the message God is trying to send us. Perhaps he doesn't want us to rely upon anything this world has to offer.

Journal Entry: June 1995

Today Amanda came into the kitchen, surprised to see me in business clothes. "Where are you going?" she asked with concern in her voice, as though I were about to abandon her. She had just assumed that since school was over I would be on summer vacation too. The tears which followed are still embedded on my collar as I write this at my office desk. I'll carry them as a badge of friendship and love today. Appearing only as a wrinkle in my shirt to those around me, they are like gold in my pocket, memories of a little girl who would rather have me by her side.

They'll also remind me of the joy in seeing Sarah comfort her sister with some "gold" of her own. Their love shall be my guide today. Their love shall keep me centered in the Lord's embrace.

Journal Entry: September 1995

This morning I asked Sarah what she wanted out of life. She thought for a while and said, "I don't know." I said, " Well, with prayer and meditation, you can have anything you'd ever want."

"But Daddy," she said, "I already have everything I'd ever want. I have you and Mommy and Amanda. God loves me and Jesus loves me. What else do I need?" And as she said that, a small tear came to her eye as if to underline the sincere and innocent nature of her wisdom. I can learn so much from her.

Where Is God in All This?

Who can truly define God? Is my God like your God? Does He look the same? Does He talk the same? Does He want the same things? Is He black or white? Is He even a he, or is He a she?

There is nothing I can offer you here that will change your perspective of your God or how you feel about Him. Only you can do that. I can't take away your anger if that's what you feel. I can't explain why God "allows" children to get sick or die. I' m not so sure myself.

What I hope to relate to you is how I believe God relates to me. How He has blessed my life. How He has shown me light where most have seen only darkness. How I find peace in the midst of the pain and how He has shown me love I could never have discovered on my own.

All I have found in the last five years has come not of my own doing. It has come to me through grace and insight of the Spirit in response to prayer for understanding. I realized a long time ago alone I can accomplish nothing. It is only by rendering myself empty and allowing the Lord to refill me can I find any answers or strength and courage to go on. It is only when I try to do things on my own I become stressed or fearful or bitter.

I suppose this chapter could be among the longest since it is potentially so controversial and in need of lengthy arguments to back up my points. However, the message is so simple I will not attempt to clutter it up with my words. I will only tell you what works for me and leave it at that. I'll defend nothing, nor will I tell you that you must choose my way of thinking to find happiness. Only you can choose what works for you. We seek the same Lord, but we all start at a different place. If it helps to add credibility to my comments, I'll tell you I've reached this place in my understanding after reading more than ten thousand pages on Eastern religions, Western religions, new age philosophy, traditional philosophy, meditation, stress management, death, life, miracles, the Bible and miscellaneous other topics too obscure to mention. I've talked with other parents in the same situation and I've talked at great length with members of the clergy about why things like this happen.

All of this was unnecessary. In the end, the answer was hidden deep within me. Only the Lord and I had the power to unlock it. I just had to take the time to listen to the still voice within me that has all the answers. But to hear that voice, I had to take a few steps, which helped to clear my mind of the clutter and noise that prevent real understanding. They helped to break down the wall we all put up to keep us in the darkness. It's the same wall that keeps the pain inside and the love outside.

For me, breaking down the wall started with the desire for understanding—*real* understanding, not quick, easy answers to questions such as, "Why does God do this to little children?" I began to need a deeper understanding of what was happening around me and why everything seemed to be crying out in such a brutal way for attention.

This need to understand took me in several directions. I prayed. I learned to meditate. I began reading everything I could find on life, death and illness. I began writing my thoughts in a journal. And I looked to the Bible, starting with the book of Job.

We've all read or heard about the story of Job, the wealthy, wise and religious man who was put through test after test at the hands of the devil. But in the end, the story of Job had more to do with how Job really felt about his Lord and himself than it did with some impulsive, cruel joke of the devil. Job's religion had become sterile and external to himself. His trials forced him to search deep within himself for true understanding and *real* faith.

I began to search inside myself for answers rather than look for something or someone to blame. And once I began to look inside, I recognized God is at the core of my very existence. I recognized within me was a spark of divinity— the same spark that exists within all of us. In this way, we are all connected. In this way, we all make up God, whether black or white, man or woman. Healthy or sick, the Lord is at our core, waiting to show all of us how to come home.

In large part, the path toward home starts with forgiveness. I truly believe forgiveness is the key to happiness. It's the magic that starts the whole process of letting go. It's the key to setting yourself free. Anger and bitterness lead only to despair and stagnation; forgiveness leads to love and growth.

For my journey home, I needed to start by forgiving myself for all the things I thought I had become. I needed to forgive my wife for all the things I felt she had done to me. I needed to forgive my innocent children for all the struggles I perceived they had put me through. And I needed to forgive my Lord for all the things I felt He had brought upon me. Not that He or anybody else needed my forgiveness—I needed to forgive them.

When I learned how to forgive, I set myself free. The need for clear-cut answers to life's questions began to melt away. I no longer needed to know who had done this to our family or why. That would only place blame, which would get me nowhere. Forgiveness took that need from me. After all, should forgiveness hold any conditions, even conditions of understanding the reason why something happens? Would you forgive your child only if you knew the reasons why he or she did something? To demand answers as a condition of forgiveness is not forgiveness at all, it's ego one-upmanship. It's a power play by the ego to demonstrate your superiority through your indiscriminate act of absolution.

Real forgiveness is unconditional. From forgiveness flows love and from love flows spirituality. But do not mistake spirituality as something you find only on a mountain top. You find it all around you, no matter where you are—whether you're on a mountain in Tibet or in the midst of a crisis on the south side of

Chicago. We do not find God by escaping the realities of our world. We find God by including Him in the realities of our world, be they joyous or tragic, exciting or routine. He is in all things, calling us all the time, leading us all back to His peace.

And so today I pray for "better" circumstances. I pray for Amanda's miraculous recovery. But I also pray to see what God is trying to show me about how to deal with her illness, about how to *live* with her illness; about how to *love* with her illness. He may never change our condition, but I *know* He has changed the way I feel about it.

As I look back, I have no more answers than when I started. I still don't know why this has happened to us. I still burn about the past. I still struggle to understand the cruelty of it all. I still fear what the eventual outcome will be. I still get angry and sad and stressed. I still feel pain. But now I've got a better idea of where to channel the pain; how to feel it and move on from it. I know there is a place inside of me where answers are not needed—a place where love and peace and stillness are found, even while the battle rages.

Perhaps my favorite part of the Bible comes in John 16:33, where Jesus says, *"These things I have spoken unto you that in me ye might have peace. In the world, ye shall have tribulation: but be of good cheer; I have overcome the world"* (King James version). In this one verse I place all my faith, hope and trust. We are not of this world, we are in it. And regardless of our circumstances in this world, we shall overcome them to return home to what we truly are—beautiful, wonderful sparks of divinity.

Because of this, I am able to look beyond Amanda's battered body and see the perfect spark of divinity that shines within her. And when I see that spark, I cannot possibly be sad about her life for in that spark lives the Lord. In that spark is a piece of me and Deborah and Sarah and you. For in that spark is my assurance I will never be completely without her, nor she without me.

I have found God in my struggle, although I am easily distracted and continually lose sight of Him. But each time I look within myself, He waits there patiently for me with the same assurances. I don't know if He will watch as Amanda's body dies, if it dies before me. But I know His love for her and for me will be perfect and unchanging, whichever way this journey ends. And in the end, that's all I need to know.

---

1. Taken from *Forgiving God* by Carla Killough McClafferty, Copyright © 1995. Used by permission of Discovery House Publishers, Box 3566, Grand Rapids MI 49501. All rights reserved.

CHAPTER 10

The Threat of Death

"I'm not so afraid of the death.
I'm afraid of the dying."

—me

Journal Entry: October 1994

It was another cool, fall morning, the kind when clouds are white on top and gray on the bottom and fly by quickly in an aggressive wind. The sky was a rich shade of blue.

Sarah and Amanda joined me on my walk with Missy, our dog. We laughed and played during this time together, skipping and hopping all the way home. We stopped at a pile of leaves and I threw them into the wind at the girls. The leaves got caught in their hair and in their coats, but mostly they danced off their faces and bodies and went flying off into the distance. Such laughter and delight from two little girls. How much fun I have with them.

In the midst of this gaiety, in between screams and laughter as the leaves brushed off their faces, little Amanda stopped and looked at me. In the most sincere voice she could provide, she said, "I like you, Daddy." Not, "I love you," which she says often, but, "I like you." Confirmation that we are friends as well as family.

In an instant, my participation in the fun ceased. I now became an observer of the moment trying desperately to capture

135

her words and her emotion into my memories, to lock them away into my thoughts where I could recall them whenever I needed to. I was afraid that I must remember Amanda, since she may not always be with me to keep me fresh with current words to lift my spirit.

And as this happened, I realized that I was seeing in slow motion. The leaves stayed in flight just a little longer. The smile on her face faded just a little more slowly. And Sarah's laughter echoed just a little more vibrantly. How I love these girls! What a treasure! What a gift!

As I watched, Sarah and Amanda returned to their play, quickly dismissing my sudden pause as an interruption to their fun. They ran off toward the house, and Missy followed. Capture the moment, Scott. Lock it away. Who knows what the world may bring you tomorrow.

Journal Entry: May 1995

Some time ago, I realized that Amanda's mission in life was to teach Deborah and me a very painful but important lesson. For me, that lesson has been love, faith, understanding and sacrifice. She has been a good teacher. I feel as though the lesson has been learned and her time to return home has come. And now I am watching my daughter die. Afraid that my resignation is part of the dying, I struggle to keep hope. Also afraid to fight nature, I struggle to find acceptance.

What is my role? Comforter to ease the transition? Or coach to keep fighting until the bitter end? They seem so mutually exclusive, with no middle ground. I could be either completely right or horribly wrong. This could be my last lesson to her. What if I fail her?

Her gift to me has been so vast, I cannot contain it in my understanding. What gift shall I provide in return? Is it spiritual or physical life? Perhaps they are not so mutually exclusive. Perhaps they are wonderfully intermixed. Perhaps in receiving her gift, I have offered her one as well.

Journal Entry: June 1995

And now her body reflects her spirit
Older than her five years would indicate
Frailty in physical form only
Strength in spirit abounds.
As her hair falls
Eyes deepen
And skin grows a yellowish pale
She looks different to me.

Even more different than
The last time we went
Through this.
Who am I looking at?

She seems resigned this time
Not given up
Not apathetic
But perhaps more prepared, more ready.

Even as I feel confident about
Her survival
I feel as though a
Surprise awaits.

A surprise for us . . .
Not for her.

The Threat of Death

I guess I realized a long time ago I could handle Amanda's death. I had envisioned it at least a hundred times. I had pictured her funeral right down to the very last detail. I could see in my mind what I was wearing and what the people looked like who came to the service. I could picture Deborah and Sarah sitting next to me. I could envision the service itself and the words that would be spoken. I even had the plans worked out for the weeks following the funeral to minimize the trauma to us all.

So when it seemed the end of her tender, young life was near, I knew it was not her actual death that bothered me. It was the process of dying I feared most. It was watching the pain and not being able to do anything about it. This has always been my greatest fear. If the end comes, how long will it take? How painful will it be?

Perhaps it's that helplessness I really fear. Isn't every father supposed to be a hero? How could I look Amanda in the eye, each of us knowing what was really happening? Would she understand I had no magic bullet? Would it be only my insecurity that would complicate the final days?

To this day, I have no answer for the best way to deal with the pending threat of my child's death. Acceptance brings me peace, but then I revert back to a fighting, never-give-up mode that refuses to accept such an end to the journey. I fear my very acceptance will be a part of what leads to her passing. I try to place it all in the hands of God, but I keep taking it back. This has been the hardest part for me to resolve. I don't know if I ever will.

I will not comment on how I will feel if Amanda ultimately succumbs to her disease. How can I really predict such a state of mind? To project my feelings at that time would be as if I wrote this book about someone else's experience in dealing with an ill child. Unless you step into it and live it, you cannot truly appreciate the depth of emotion and the impact it has on your everyday life.

But I can tell you about how I was feeling at the moment I thought Amanda actually was going to die. One night not long ago, I was absolutely convinced she would be dead before morning. We had been up with her for four hours and on more than one occasion she had actually stopped breathing. But each time, she would spring back after about thirty seconds and start screaming again about the pain.

When she finally lost consciousness about 2 A.M., we laid her back on her bed and stared at her for an hour. When we could see that she was still breathing, I took my notepad and began to write her eulogy. I knew when she died I would not be able to function very well and I wanted to write down what I thought about Amanda's life, as well as her premature death.

These are the words that came flowing out of me:

Some of you might believe that Amanda's life has been a tragedy, seemingly endless years of needless suffering for a child who deserved so much better. And if you look at her life in a vacuum, you'd be right.

But the real tragedy would be to look at her life and not understand its purpose. How many people go through their lives wondering why they're here? Wondering if they've ever made a difference or if they ever will?

Well, Amanda has given me the gift of knowing not only what her life has been all about, but mine as well. The lessons were hidden in the years of despair and pain, but they were speaking volumes each and every day.

Amanda came into this world for many reasons, but I know that part of why she came here was for me. Her unselfish gift of the spirit was to bring joy into my life. Her lessons were about love without conditions, hope in the midst of despair, courage in the middle of the storm and faith in the Lord our God, no matter what our trials might be. I never would have learned any of these lessons to the depth that I have today without her as my mentor.

I'd also suggest that she has come here for her mother and sister, who will love Amanda deeply for eternity. Her lessons certainly did not stop at the boundaries of my body, but extend to this day to Deborah and Sarah, as well as to our family, friends, neighbors and many others. Some of these people have never even seen her, but share her pain through anyone who has ever told her story. Our lives were blessed through their gift of prayer for a child who needed it, as well as support for her parents, who needed help too.

*And now my life. What am I here for? My purpose was—
and is—to respond to the trial; to learn to serve, not lead; to
learn to give and find pure joy in the giving; to learn to share
my feelings with those around me; to accept support from
family and friends and find no shame in not being able to
stand alone; to trust the Lord and find His peace, even in
turmoil; to be a witness for hope; to forgive the Lord for what
seems to be unjust punishment. (The Lord does not need our
forgiveness, but He wants it.)*

*My friends, there are no wasted lives, only unlearned les-
sons. I am grateful that I have been able to identify one of
my teachers. I will spend the rest of my life striving to live the
example Amanda has set for me.*

*To find strength, I will look not only to Amanda, but to
Deborah and Sarah, all of you, and the Lord. I know not if
I have passed—or will yet pass—the trial set before me. I
only know that failure will come only if I do not try. Only if
I do not believe that I can succeed.*

*Do not be bitter about Amanda's life. Find joy in it! Think of
the gift we all have received in knowing her, in loving her.
She is a special child with an ancient wisdom. When I grow
up, I want to be just like her.*

Today, even though I am able to think so much more about
her life than her death, it's amazing how quickly and easily I fall
back into the trap. Just this morning she came down stairs bent
over, complaining of severe stomach pain. Within five seconds, I
relived her whole life, death and funeral. It's almost automatic
for me.

The good news is I'm now able to recognize what I'm doing and move on. The bad news is I don't get too far. As I approach
the day today, I know what I'll think about more than anything
else—am I watching my daughter die?

EPILOGUE

> *"There is only one reason why I am here today. What kept me alive was you. Others gave up hope. I dreamed that some day I would be here telling you how I , Viktor Frankl, had survived Nazi concentration camps. I've never been here before, I've never seen any of you before, I've never given this speech before. But in my dreams I have stood before you and said these words a thousand times."*
>
> —Viktor Frankl[1]

It is entirely possible writing this book was as much about helping me as it was about helping others. It served three purposes for me.

First, writing it helped me express myself and explore the deepest realms of what I was feeling about Amanda. I'm not sure I processed all that had happened until I was forced to write about it. On more than one occasion I had to stop writing because the pain was too deep. But it was that same pain that allowed me to exorcize the last of my anger and bitterness, at least for now.

141

Second, this book is what kept me sane during many difficult days and nights. The passion for writing it helped me focus
my energy on something positive. It provided a goal and helped
me find something good out of all the tragedy. Maybe, just maybe,
this book was the answer as to why Amanda got sick in the first
place—so that she could serve as an example for other families
trying to endure and overcome tragedy.

And last, the book also became a way in which I could see
Amanda as part of my future and not just my past. In the early
stages of her illness, I used to envision Amanda walking down
the aisle on her wedding day. It was a statement of hope to myself she was going to be OK, but as time went on I lowered my
expectations and envisioned her graduating from high school.
Then as things got really bad, I began to envision this book. I'd
picture in my mind the story of hope I could recount as Amanda
made it through yet another death sentence. I pictured her turning seven when the book was finished. She had to be alive for
the story to work. It was my way to hold on to her for just a
while longer. I'd worry about her turning eight later, on after the
book was published.

As I read back over these pages, I'm amazed at what I've
written. I can't believe I've shared so much about my feelings. I
am not an expressive person. I tend to be quiet and reserved
about all things, especially Amanda. My friends will undoubt-
edly be equally astonished at the depth of my emotion.

Even my wife was often surprised to read my thoughts as
she scanned early drafts of the book. My family also learned
more about how I've dealt with Amanda's illness from reading
the drafts than they ever got from anything I've said. But as
with everything, there is a reason. My journey would not have
been complete without going through this process, and learning
how to share and be more open.

Amanda is doing very well, I am delighted to report. It is
now over a year since I first sat down at the computer to write

my introduction. We've had several scares and some difficult times as a family during the last twelve months, but all in all, this has been the best year out of the last five. We've had some time to assimilate all that's happened to us and accept it for what it is.

We came within days of losing one of our greatest treasures and today she stands before us a playful, delightful child. As the treatments have become a bit more routine, Amanda's personality has truly blossomed. It turns out she's a very happy child, something we didn't know before. She's also become very popular at school despite a rough start with a bald head, and she has developed some very close friends who love her dearly.

Perhaps the best description of her personality can be found in a single story:

We recently took a wonderful trip to Disney World sponsored by the Make-A-Wish Foundation and Give Kids the World, two incredibly generous organizations I encourage you to support. Mickey Mouse appeared and was walking down the street. With great excitement I exclaimed to Amanda and Sarah in a very loud voice, "Mickey is here! Mickey is here!"

Amanda turned and looked at me with a little disgust in her expression and said, "Daddy, it's just a guy in a suit." And with that, she and Sarah took off and waited for hugs and kisses and pictures with "the suit." As we watched, I saw all that life has to offer unfold before me. I saw joy, excitement, fantasy and dreams. I also saw a touch of the loss of innocence and the recognition not everything is as wonderful as it's cracked up to be. But even with that, I saw how the heart of a child can still find love and faith.

If Amanda can do that, maybe I can still picture her walking down the aisle on her wedding day. When the time comes, you'll have no idea how proud I'll feel to be just another "guy in a suit." I can only hope I get as many hugs and kisses and pictures as Mickey.

May God bless you and keep you all the days of your lives. Amen.

---

1. John C. Maxwell on Viktor Frankl, *Developing the Leader Within You*, Copyright © 1993, Thomas Nelson, Inc., Nashville, TN, p.159.

2. Tian Dayton, Ph.D. on Arthur Rubenstein, *The Quiet Voice of the Soul*, Copyright © 1995, Health Communications, Deerfield Beach, FL, p.199,

RECOMMENDED READING

I have read many, many books on illness, death, hope and spirituality. My original goal for reading them was to find some answers. I found none. My secondary goal was to find something to help me handle the day-to-day stress. Here I was partly successful. My final goal was to open my mind to help me find the answers myself. Here I was very successful.

Many of the books I read were not soothing at all. They challenged my thinking and made me very uncomfortable. Many of them made me angry or went contrary to traditional religious teaching. Many of them were "way out there" and strange.

But in the end, these books allowed me to expand my thinking and find a new way of looking at Amanda's illness. Many of them encouraged me to look within myself for answers, which is where I ultimately found peace.

For this section, however, I will recommend those books that offer more "practical" advice on dealing with serious illness and death. I'll also recommend only a few books because I want this section to be helpful, not an intimidating list that turns into more of an exercise, ultimately leading to more stress.

Reading List

Foundation For Inner Peace. *A Course In Miracles*. Glen Ellen: 1975, 1985, 1992. A long study in spirituality, that requires more than a year's investment in time. There is a great deal of discussion on health and illness that offered me a very different perspective from more traditional teachings. I'm not sure if I agree with its new-age approach, but the writing is beautiful and so is its message. This book helped me get through some of the darkest times but don't start it if you aren't prepared to open your mind and invest a lot of time.

Gunther, John. *Death Be Not Proud*. New York: Harper and Row Publishers, Inc. 1949. This is a memoir a father wrote of his son who died after a lengthy battle with a brain tumor. Although it is an older book, it's relevant to today's parental struggles.

Hirshberg, Caryle, and Mark Ian Barasch *Remarkable Recovery*. New York: Riverhead Books, 1995 The premise of this book is we should study more aggressively the reasons some people go into spontaneous remission, rather than cast off their recoveries as an anomaly Perhaps some important answers to major health issues await us if we would only take the time to look at how the body heals itself.

Komp, Diane M., M.D. *A Window to Heaven*. Grand Rapids: Zondervan Publishing House, 1992. Dr. Komp is a Christian physician who believes in both the physical and spiritual aspects of healing.

Komp, Daine M., M.D. *A Child Shall Lead Them*. Grand Rapids: Zondervan Publishing House, 1993. Dr. Komp chronicles the story of a little girl who becomes the first child to receive a bone marrow transplant. This girl has the same illness as Amanda.

Krementz, Jill. *How it Feels to Fight for Your Life*. Boxton: Little, Brown and Company, Inc., 1989. This is a collection of stories of young heroes who find hope despite their serious illnesses.

Kubler-Ross, Elisabeth. *On Death and Dying*. New York: Macmillan Publishing Co., 1969. This is a great book for those struggling with the concept of death. It may also be particularly useful for those with older children. This is the book that out-lines the stages leading to acceptance I reference in Chapter One.

Kubler-Ross, Elisabeth. *On Children and Death*. New York: Macmillan Publishing Company, 1983. I highly recommend this book for any parent with a seriously ill child. Dr. Ross's book deals more with life than with death and is filled with beautiful writing from children and parents alike.

Maier, Frank. *Sweet Reprieve*. New York: Crown Publishers, Inc., 1991. A well-told story written by a *Newsweek* journalist who suffers from heart and liver disease that ultimately lead to a liver transplant. He speaks not only of his illness but how it impacted his life and the lives of those around him. His per-spective is one of hope and I would highly recommend his book. You'll need to look for it in the library as it is no longer in print.

McClafferty, Carla Killough. *Forgiving God*. Grand Rapids: Dis-covery House Publishers, 1995. This is a Christian book about a woman whose son is killed on a swing set. Her search for an-swers is very touching.

Parkhill, Steven C. *Answer Cancer*. Deerfield Beach: Health Com-munications, Inc. 1995. This is an alternative look at the answer to cancer. This has a spiritual approach that may not be appreci-ated by all readers, but it will open your mind.

Prather, Hugh and Gayle. *I Will Never Leave You*. New York: Bantam Books, 1995. This is the book I recommended in Chap-ter Seven. It's a terrific guide to finding strength and love in your marriage.

Schiff, Harriet Sarnoff. *The Bereaved Parent*. New York: Penguin Books, 1978. This is a book written by a mother who lost her son to illness. It discusses the after-effects of his death and how it impacted her entire family. If you have lost your child, you may wish to read this one.

Siegel, Bernie S., M.D. *Love, Medicine and Miracles.* New York: Harper and Row, Publishers, 1986. This would be a great first book for you to read. Dr. Siegel was one of the pioneers of his profession to add love, spirituality, humanity and tenderness to his practice of modern medicine. He believes in the scientific and spiritual aspects of healing.

Sorteberg, Leanne, with Lisa C. Ragsdale. *Your Child Doesn't Have to Die.* Burnsville, MN: Abundant Living Press, 1996. A wonderful story written by a mother who chooses to treat her son (successfully) through nutritional therapy. This book was self-published, and you can contact the author at abundiv@aol.com or PO Box 1092, Burnsville, MN 55337.

The Holy Bible. Pick up any version! Christ's answers are written in the Bible's pages.

A REQUEST

Amanda's primary illness is called Langerhan's cell histio-cytosis. Histio is a very rare disease that receives no public funding for research. Consequently, we must fund all research with private donations.

If you can afford to make a contribution, please do so. Checks can be made out to the Histiocytosis Association of America and mailed to the following address:

Histiocytosis Association of America
302 North Broadway
Pitman, NJ 08071

If you would like, you can make this donation in honor of Amanda MacLellan.

All funds go toward research and education on histiocyto-sis. Parents of children with histio also receive valuable information on the disease, which helps them to better understand the nature and circumstance of the illness.

Thank you.

*"Most people ask for happiness on condition
Happiness can only be felt if you
don't set any condition."*

—Arthur Rubenstein[1]

BIBLIOGRAPHY

Dayton, Tian Ph.D. *The Quiet Voice of the Soul*. Deerfield Beach, FL: Health Communications, 1995.

Komp, Diane M., M.D. *A Child Shall Lead Them*. Grand Rapids, MI: Zondervan Publishing House, 1992.

Komp, Diane M., M.D., *A Window to Heaven*. Grand Rapids, MI: Zondervan Publishing House, 1992.

Kubler-Ross, Elisabeth. *On Death and Dying*. New York: Macmillan Publishing Co., 1969, 1993, 1997.

Kubler-Ross, Elisabeth. *On Children and Death*. New York: Macmillan Publishing Company, 1983, 1993, 1997.

Maxwell, John C. *Developing the Leader Within You*. Nashville, TN: Thomas Nelson, 1993.

McClafferty, Carla Killough. *Forgiving God*. Grand Rapids, MI: Discovery House Publishers, 1995.

Give the Hope of *Amanda's Gift* to Your Friends and Loved Ones

CHECK YOUR LEADING BOOKSTORE OR ORDER HERE

❑ **YES**, I want _____ copies of *Amanda's Gift* at $12.95 each, plus $3 shipping per book (Georgia residents please add $.91 sales tax per book). Canadian orders must be accompanied by a postal money order in U.S. funds. Allow 15 days for delivery.

My check or money order for $_____ is enclosed.

Name _____

Organization _____

Address _____

City/State/Zip _____

Phone _____

Please make your check payable and return to:

Health Awareness Communications

215 Spearfield Trace

Roswell, GA 30075